A Journey

FROM SUNSHINE
TO SHADOW

PARIS L. BUMP

DORRANCE
PUBLISHING CO
EST. 1920
PITTSBURGH, PENNSYLVANIA 15238

Dorrance Publishing Co
585 Alpha Drive
Suite 103
Pittsburgh, PA 15238
Visit our website at *www.dorrancebookstore.com*

ISBN: 978-1-6853-7035-0
EISBN: 978-1-6853-7885-1

A Journey

FROM SUNSHINE
TO SHADOW

THE JOURNEY
FROM
SUNSHINE TO SHADOW

There are many enemies of the mind.
The most insidious invades without warning.
And slowly takes a precious life from
sunshine into deepening shadow.

It is called Alzheimer's disease.

To date, there is no known cure.

TABLE OF CONTENTS

DEDICATION

This book is dedicated to the many selfless caregivers who toil night and day providing for the needs of someone suffering through the debilitating stages of Alzheimer's disease.

All elements of this book are protected and cannot be duplicated or used
without consent of the author.

INTRODUCTION

The accounts contained in this book are intended to provide the reader with an image of the tragic and painful journey travelled by a victim of Alzheimer's and to the loved ones who witnessed the slow decline and final days of her life.

The general public knows little about Alzheimer's and even less about why so little funding and research is devoted to its prevention and cure. Considering the rapid aging and demographics of the population, it should be obvious that public funding for this disease is grossly inadequate.

The onset of Alzheimer's disease is moving down the age ladder. Some cases have been recorded of victims in their early thirties and an increasing number of the afflicted fall into the 45–55 age range—and that should demand more attention and action.

The brilliant woman portrayed in this book was afflicted at age sixty-four and passed away two months short of her seventy-first birthday.

Without the help and support of the several loyal women who provided care and assistance through the years of suffering and anguish endured by this dear woman, the toll on the author would have been unbearable.

There are more good and kind people around us than we realize—more than some would have us believe.

PART 1

Chapter One

BEGINNING A BEAUTIFUL JOURNEY

On a hot June day in 1973, I had the honor of giving the keynote speech in Zurich for the International Quality Control Conference. When I concluded, I rushed to the hotel's penthouse lounge to wet my pipes and found the local executive secretary club meeting had just ended and some of its members were there dancing and drinking. One of my companions nudged me and commented.

"These women are the best you'll find between here and Geneva. I mean in terms of their professional competence, of course."

I sipped a cold beer and quietly watched the action until a tall blonde with shoulder-length hair captured my attention. I asked my companion if he knew who she was.

"Oh yeah, I met her once. It was at the airport, as I remember. At the time, she was the personal secretary of a CEO at a big company here in Zurich."

I asked if that was all he knew about her.

"Well, she's also head of the executive secretary's association in Zurich. I think her name is Anita, but I'm not sure."

When the music stopped, I walked to the bar where she was talking with her lady friends. I introduced myself and asked if she would like to dance. She hesitated, looked me over, and at first, I thought she didn't like what she saw, but she flashed a bright smile and accepted. We danced a few times and then talked for an hour at a table overlooking the city. It was a dance that would last forty-five, unforgettable, love-filled years.

Finding each other

I learned that Anita was the daughter of a resort hotel owner in the town of Pontresina in the Engadine valley, a few miles from St. Moritz. She and her family were well known in the valley and when in her teens, on one Swiss national day, she had been dubbed "Jewel of the Valley."

Anita was the oldest daughter of the family and, as dictated by local custom, could wear the traditional costume of Canton Chur.

Anita lived in a studio apartment in Zurich's Old City (Altstadt) on the south side of Prediger Platz, a small park rimmed by coffee shops, bookshops, small boutiques, and the city library. It was a short tram ride to her office and convenient to the shops and restaurants she frequented. She had many friends and coworkers and worked out three or four times a week at her fitness club. Her attention to fitness showed in her appearance.

For my part, I was living in a large apartment in Brussels. Mainly due to my ex-wife having taken away all the household things that suited her when she left, the place was very spartan. Although I could cook, I rarely used the kitchen. Considering I was in the midst of some of the finest eating places in Europe, it was silly not to take advantage of them. I made an effort at my appearance and had a good tailor in Brussels and one in London.

My office was two miles from the apartment and by forcing myself to walk there and back in good weather, together with bike riding and jogging in the nearby parks, I could keep my weight under control. Too many plane rides and sitting through long meetings were the enemies of fitness.

On the first weekend after we met, I flew to Zurich to see Anita. I hadn't expected her to be at the airport, but she was there.

"Anita, you didn't have to come all the way out here."

She smiled and patted my hand.

"That's our custom when a friend visits."

I couldn't take my eyes off her. She was wearing a black pantsuit with a gold and brown Hermès scarf and looked taller than when we first met. I looked down, expecting her to be in high heels, but she was wearing casual loafers. I was a six-footer and if she had been in high heels, I might not have been the taller. Every aspect of her continued to command my attention.

The train arrived for the city and she asked about the weather in Brussels.

"The Belgians who come to our hotel in Pontresina say there is more rain in Brussels than sunshine. Is that true?"

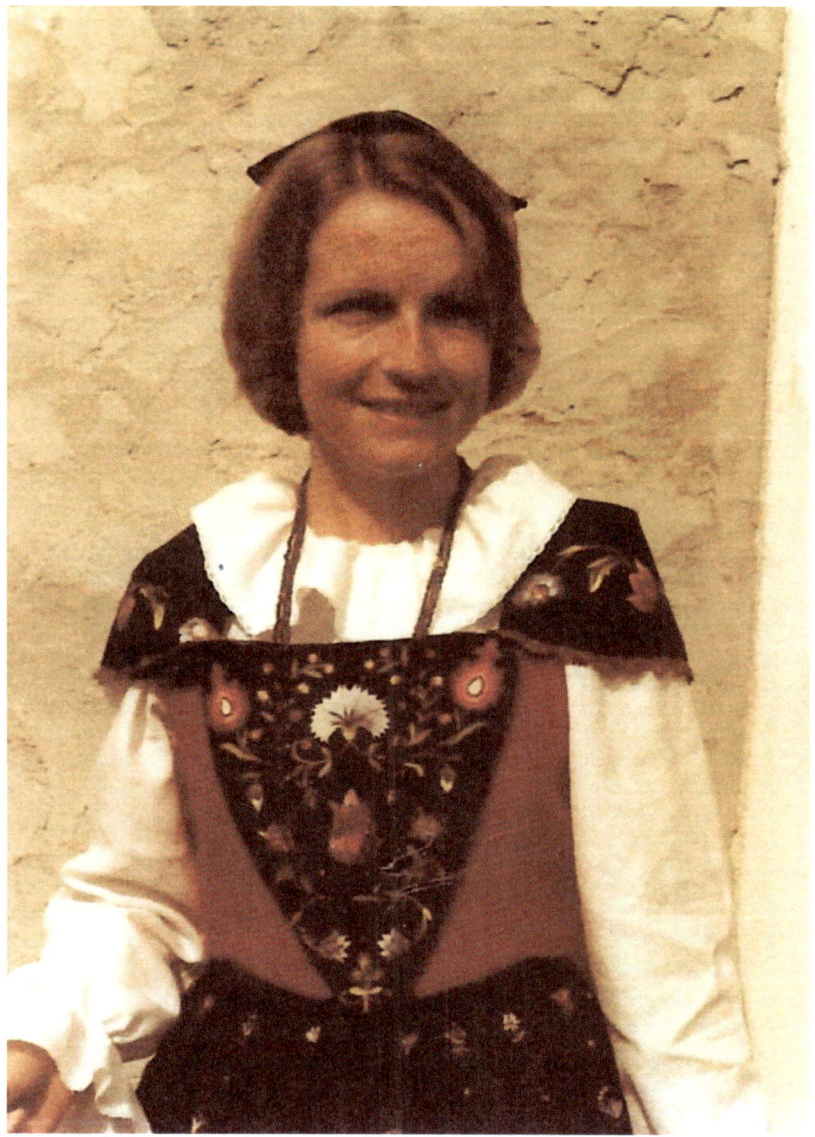

Anita Merkt in Engadine National Costume – 1963
As the oldest daughter, she wore this handmade costume for cantonal
and national holidays.

I admitted the sky was clear only about twenty percent of the year. I told her I travelled outside Belgium most of the time, so it didn't really bother me.

It turned out to be a warm and exciting weekend, and Anita had been all that I dreamed she would be. She was cultured and intelligent, spoke six languages, and had an open sense of humor. We agreed to give our relationship three months to mature, before making any deep commitment.

Three months passed quickly and our relationship became stronger each day. I met the Merkt family and friends in Pontresina and was warmly received by all—with one exception—her father's dog, Oscar, an avalanche dog trained for searches in the snow—he growled when I approached him. Gustaf Merkt was a mountain guide and head of the mountain search and avalanche rescue team for the area and he loved Oscar. I knew I had to make friends with him.

Bernina Haus, the family hotel, was situated on the north side of the Bernina pass at the foot of the Diavolezza ski area. The family had once owned the small ski lodge at the top of the area overlooking the Bernina glacier. Anita had worked in the lodge in her early teens, selling candy and cigarettes to the skiers. She told me she had to lead a pair of mules loaded with supplies up the mountain each week and was thankful when her parents sold the lodge.

When we had some quiet moments together, she told me of her childhood in Pontresina.

"We have a lot of snow in this area and often the train couldn't get to our hotel, so my sisters and I had to ski down to school in the village. If the plow train hadn't opened the pass, we had to stay overnight in the village with a family who owned a small café with rooms for skiers. That was always fun."

The mountain, La Galp, was a quarter mile up the pass from the hotel and was a practice slope for the Swiss national ski team. The slope was too tough for me, but Anita said she had managed it a few times without breaking any bones. She knew I was no daredevil on skis, so we never ventured beyond the modest slopes of St. Moritz.

When waiting for my flight back to Belgium, I asked Anita if she would consider moving to Brussels.

"Paris, it's too soon to make that decision. I don't rule it out, but there is too much to be considered at this stage."

I had been hopeful, but wasn't surprised by her reply and knew the eighteen-year age difference was a major factor.

I told her she was right and we did need more time to be sure our relationship allowed such a commitment. I agreed we should hold the thought for a few more months.

She gave a little smile of relief.

"Yes, I know we agreed to wait three months before making any major decision, and these last three months have been wonderful, but I need a little more time. Let's just see what happens."

With the matter on hold, I promised to fly down to Zurich each weekend.

Two months later, Anita called and said she agreed to live with me in Brussels, but had to spend a month wrapping up loose ends in Zurich.

I was so happy, it put a fixed smile on my face that baffled my colleagues. They would soon meet the reason for the smile.

It took me a week to find a new apartment in the Auderghem Suburb of Brussels. Two weeks later, I rented a van, drove to Zurich, packed and loaded her things, and we headed to Belgium to begin a happy and lasting life together.

Anita wore a blue silk gown for our first night in Auderghem. Her long blonde hair and blue eyes were captivating and I was struck dumb as we sat before the fireplace.

After a dinner we had prepared together, I kicked myself for having forgotten to buy film for my camera. It was an unforgettable night that should have been recorded.

We were up early for breakfast and I asked about her plans for the day.

"I'm not traveling this week, so maybe tonight we can roam the old city and the Grand Place to find a nice place to eat."

"Don't worry, Cheri. I'll spend time here arranging things—you know, making things nice and orderly.

That set me back for a moment.

"What does nice and orderly mean? Never mind. I know I'm a lousy housekeeper."

She kissed me, laughed, and pushed me out the door.

"Adieu, Paris. Have a nice day and eat a good lunch. A special dinner will be ready here by seven o'clock."

I took the tram to Brussels and left the car for her to use for shopping and exploring.

Chapter Two

MAKING THE COMMITMENT

Anita's family had taken to calling me Parigi, the Italian version of Paris. I didn't mind, and it stuck with me for the remainder of our life together.

In September of 1975, we decided to fly to Las Vegas and get married. Anita didn't want a big wedding and the Las Vegas solution suited her, but it caused some problems back in Pontresina when we returned and our reception was joyful for everyone but her father. Her mother took us aside and told us why.

"Papa is disappointed because he couldn't give his oldest daughter a big wedding at home. He feels it has hurt his standing in the village."

Anita said she thought it was also because we hadn't first asked for his blessing.

"He often talked about throwing a big party for me when the time came to get harnessed."

Her mother said he was also concerned about the eighteen-year age difference.

Several months passed before Gustaf Merkt fully accepted the marriage and me as his capable new son-in-law. Anita was much relieved that I was now included in most family discussions.

During our first seven years, we made two trips to Rio and Sao Paulo, Brazil. I told Anita it was a long business trip I didn't much like to make twice a year. She reacted as I expected she would.

"Oh, Parigi. Don't say that. These Brazilians are wonderful. They always have a smile—even the poorest. We see smiles on the street everywhere. I love that wherever we go in the city at night there are roaming samba bands. The whole city seems always to be dancing."

Anita was ever upbeat and positive, one of the many things I loved about her.

We made an annual trip to Innsbruck, Austria to visit Werner Miacher, an old friend from my days in Libya. Anita's favorite dessert was apple strudel and she had it every day we were in Innsbruck. Gudrun,

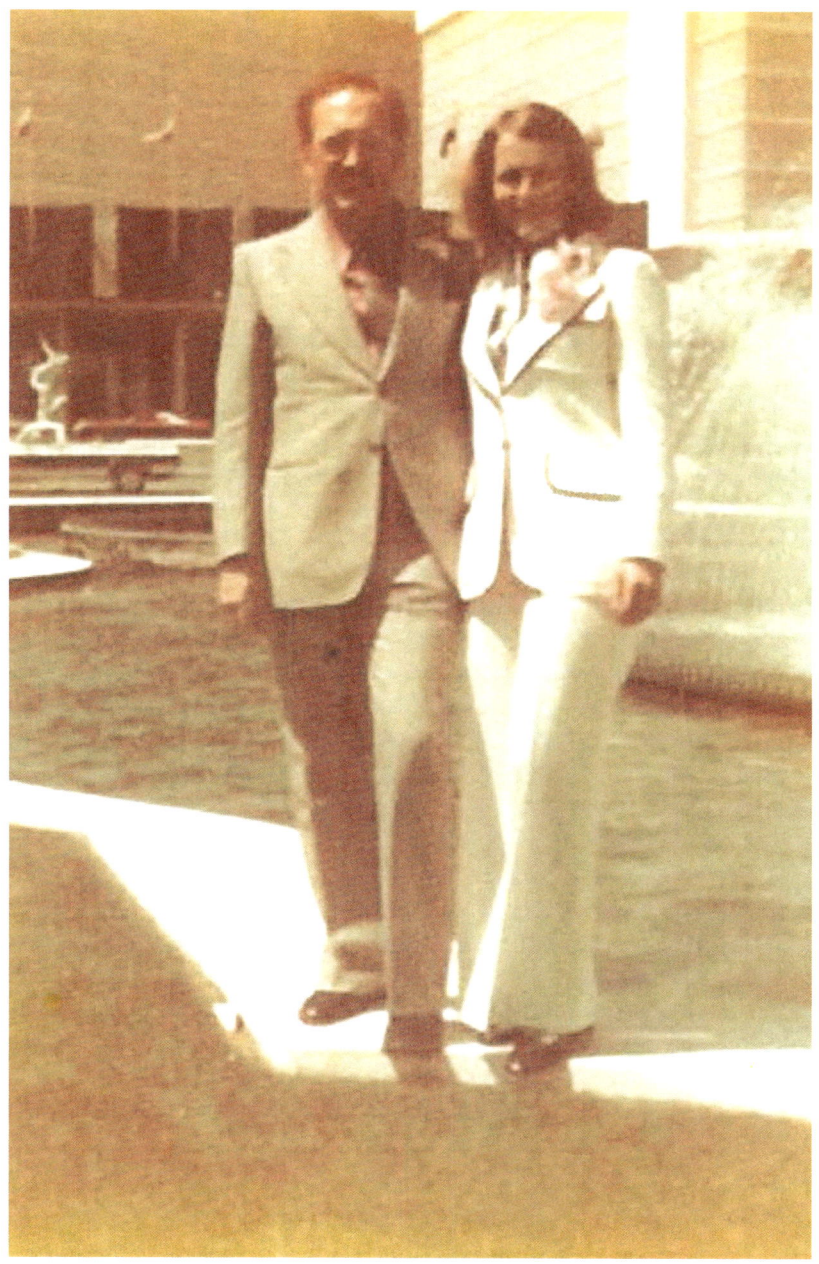

On our wedding day in Las Vegas – 1975

his wife, would remark about Anita's appetite. "It amazes me how she can eat so well and never gain weight."

In Brussels, Anita joined a riding club in the Bois de la Cambre, the nearby city park. She laughed when I asked what she did there. "We ride for an hour, have lunch, drink champagne and brag about our husbands."

In early 1976, I left Brussels for a new position in Paris and Anita was thrilled with the idea of living in her favorite city. Our apartment was in Circle Foch, just south of the Arch of Triumph. Anita soon new most of the residents.

"Parigi. Do you know who lives in this building with us?

"No, I don't."

"Sophia Lauren is on the fourth floor, Klaus Kinski is on the third, Omar Sharif and the son of the Cuban dictator are on the second. Batista lives right above us. Oh, I forgot. The sister of the Shah of Iran lives directly across from us on avenue Foch."

Now I knew why we had so much security.

Anita enrolled in a top fashion design studio for ten months of classes and earned a much-prized certificate. Most of our free time was spent exploring museums, shopping in famous boutiques, and eating in top restaurants, bistros, and sidewalk cafés. We were extremely happy and Anita glowed like a teenager from morning till night. She took the cue from a woman at the fashion studio and had her hair dyed and re-styled. It was a new look that drew only compliments.

The joy of our life in Paris was soon to be interrupted by a new opportunity. One that appeared out of the blue, one that brought a major change in our lives and careers.

In December of 1977, I was approached by a management recruiter from a New York-based consulting firm searching Europe for someone capable of turning around the Europe operations of an American company. The position was in Geneva, Switzerland. I told Anita about the opportunity and she reacted like the trooper she was.

"It sounds like another good career opportunity, Parigi. You should find out more about it."

I worried about uprooting her from the city she loved, but at least she would be in the beautiful, French-speaking area of Lake Geneva.

After two meetings in Geneva, I found the new challenge and the pay was too good to turn down, so I accepted.

Anita arranged and supervised our move from Paris to a luxurious villa apartment in Lussy-sur-Morges, near Lausanne on Lake Geneva. I saw a hint of sadness as she packed our things. I held her in my arms and assured her we would come back to Paris many times in the coming years. She patted my cheek in loving tenderness.

"Parigi, we only live once. Think of the beautiful memories we have of our life in Paris—I know I will."

Of course, she was right. Everywhere we went and each thing we enjoyed together provided another stone for the golden pyramid of memories we were building together.

Starting another chapter in our lives

I arranged for a three-week delay before starting my new job in Geneva. We both wanted some time for visiting places we both enjoyed.

We drove to Zurich to spend a day with friends, before driving south and over the Gotthard Pass to Lake Como. The Alpine peaks were still white, but Como was warm and inviting. We checked into a small hotel in the city center and Anita was anxious to prowl the famous silk shops for additions to her wardrobe. In spite of my resistance, she insisted that I buy some silk ties and suit-pocket handkerchiefs.

"Anita, these ties cost twice as much as any sane man should spend on himself."

"Parigi, these are handmade, one-of-a-kind silk ties and kerchiefs. You know you are a snappy dresser and always stand out in a crowd. These are nice assets for your wardrobe."

We visited the plush hotels along the west side of the lake and rummaged through their boutiques before settling down to a very expensive lunch. In such settings, lunch never took less than two hours, but it was well worth the time spent. Anita made the setting more radiant and was served with grace by the dining room staff—her Italian was impeccable and she always stole the show.

After two days, we left Como and drove south to Forte dei Marmi on the Italian west coast. Each year the Merkt family had spent the month of May in this quaint town while their hotel, as most hotels in Pontresina and St. Moritz, closed for a month.

We stayed at a family hotel near the beach and rented two bicycles—getting around the village was easier on two wheels because the streets were very narrow and parking places limited. The beautiful, white sand beach stretched for two miles and bikes were essential for us to visit Anita's favorite beach club restaurants. Anita was always ahead and motioning for me to catch up—her physical fitness was showing, much to my chagrin.

Our favorite restaurant was on the edge of the town square. It was owned by Alberto Corrupt, a well-known artist and master chef.

We were always well received by Alberto and eager to try his daily special and, because of Anita's sparkling personality, we had more than one free lunch there.

For the two years, until the profit turnaround I was hired for was complete, we lived in the quaint village Lussy-sur-Morges on the edge of Lake Geneva near Lausanne. With the help of several of the group's company managers, the European group of the company was brought from a six-million-dollar loss to a seven-million-dollar profit. My employment contract brought me an eight percent share of the turnaround and an opportunity to start a business of my own. Because the mother company was family-owned, I knew there was little chance of me rising in the management, so I put in my resignation.

Over the two years we were in Morges, we made several friends. The owner of our villa apartment in Lussy-sur-Morges was Madam Astor, the ex-wife of one of the Astor family, who was also a member of the family that owned the Lindt chocolate company.

Madam Astor was a friend of Oona Chaplin, Charley Chaplin's widow, and Audrey Hepburn. Hepburn owned a large villa just down the hill from Astor's place.

On several occasions, Anita joined Madam Astor and Audrey Hepburn for lunch at the boutique coffee shop and bakery in Morges center. I never asked Anita what they talked about when they were together.

Oona Chaplin was a friend and golfing companion of Madam Astor and Anita had joined them at the golf course on two occasions. She said her performance had not been as bad as predicted.

I knew breaking these remarkable social ties would be difficult for Anita, but she was always eager for a new adventure and was supportive of my proposal to move to Zurich as headquarters for my fledgling consulting business. I knew we would make weekend trips to Morges during the year.

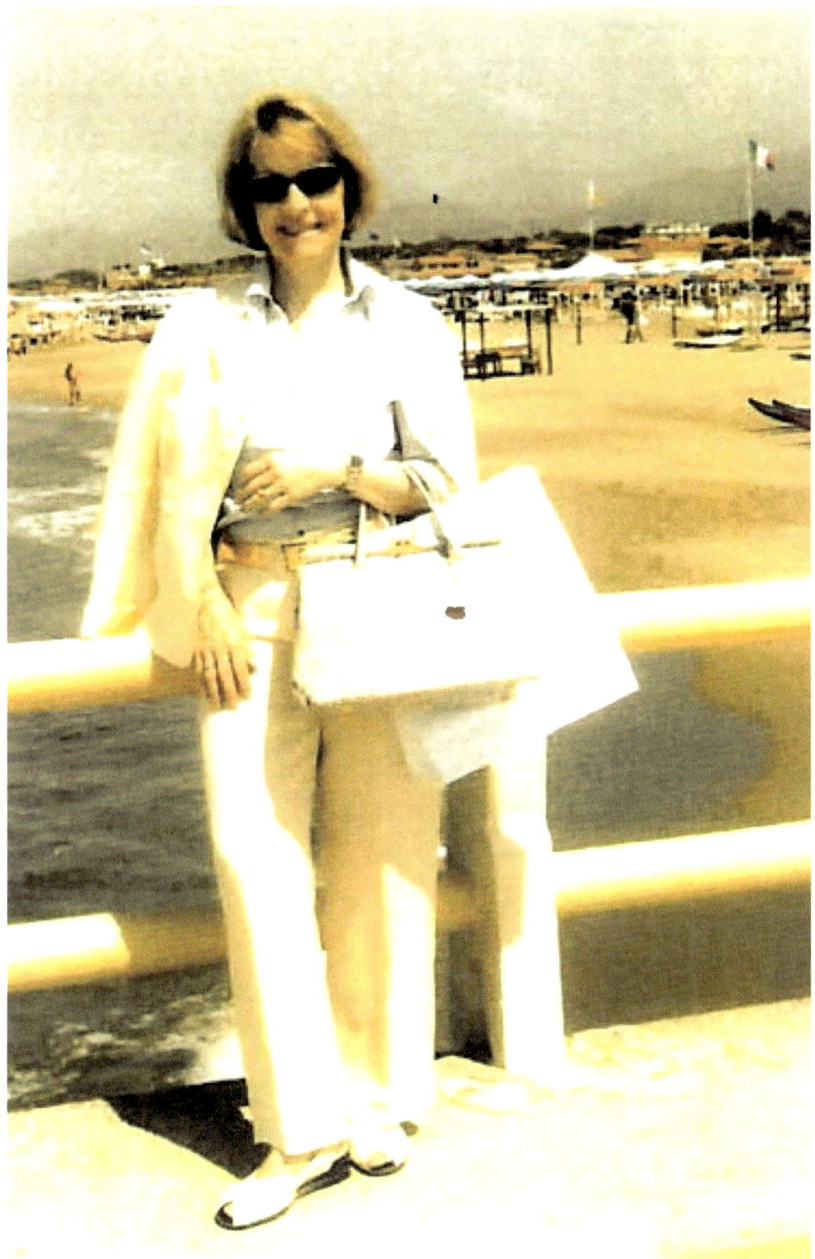

Anita at the beach in Forte dei Marmi

PART II

Chapter Three

TWO NEW CAREERS

By May of 1980, we were settled in Zurich and we named our company BERKT Management. The B was for Bump and the ERKT was for Anita's family name. My answer when asked about the name choice: "It catches your attention."

Anita was indispensable as company office manager, and with her help, we landed our first client—a well-known Swiss truck maker. We were promoting ourselves as specialists in automotive market research and new technology applications.

The Zurich location was chosen because it was smack dab in the middle of Europe and within easy driving distance to twenty vehicle builders and to over one hundred automotive component suppliers and meant our air travel costs would be minimal. In addition, all our targeted Asian automakers had both technical and market research centers in Europe.

In November 1981, Anita said she had learned of an interesting job opening as the executive secretary to a top director at the largest bank in Zurich and told me she was going to look into it. Within a week, she landed the position.

"Parigi, you will soon be running around Europe half the time, so now I want to start my own career—in banking, not in consulting. Women are beginning to get ahead in the Swiss banking world. It's not as chauvinistic as it was ten years ago, so I think I can get ahead."

She said she had found a highly qualified replacement for herself. It was Frau Oehler, a highly qualified woman Anita had known since 1972.

The thought of Anita not being at my side each day was hard to imagine, but her happiness was of utmost importance to me. I assured her that if things didn't turn out at the bank, she would always have a senior place at BERKT.

She handed her duties over to the extremely capable Frau Margrit Oehler. Margrit spoke four languages, was adept at all office technologies, and served me unfailingly for twenty years. She has remained a close friend to us both.

Over the next five years, we built a successful consulting service staffed by early retirees from the automotive and high-tech industries. Each consultant worked on a project-by-project basis for projects of anywhere from two months to eight months' duration. These highly experienced colleagues were enthusiastic and pleased with both their fees and the use of large chunks of free time between projects to travel and enjoy favorite activities.

Our clients were impressed by the experience and knowledge of the BERKT group, and we soon earned a high reputation among auto industry companies in Europe, America, and Japan. As our number of client projects grew, so did the number of highly qualified applicants who were eager to work with us.

Anita also made rapid progress in her career. Her reputation for organizational insight and problem-solving was quickly recognized by upper echelons of the bank. As expected, she stood out at every business and social gathering and quickly became the benchmark for her friends and her fellow bank employees.

On Saturdays, we walked along the lakeside to Bahnhofstrasse in Zurich where we did some shopping and often met one or two bank directors who stopped to talk and often joined us for coffee or lunch. Wherever we went, she was the center of attraction and I realized she was my greatest asset.

In 1983 we decided our Zurich apartment was inadequate for two career professionals and moved to a larger apartment in Zollikon, an upscale village one kilometer south on the lake. Apartments in Zollikon were in high demand but with recommendations to the landlord from a senior bank officer, Anita secured a long-term lease arrangement.

Once again, I was proud of what Anita could do in the face of difficult odds. She had found us a lovely home that lasted us for over twenty-five years, a home where we welcomed many prominent guests and many dear friends and relatives.

I brought my cooking skills to play each Thanksgiving and Christmas when we put on an elaborate feast for our local friends. The favorite toppers were homemade apple and pumpkin pies.

Anita was an outstanding and popular woman with many friends in Zurich and our new home village of Zollikon, but she was mostly known by her female friends and colleagues for her annual Hen Party. This was a dinner she gave at our home consisting of melted raclette cheese, wine, and champagne consumed amid a stream of jokes about

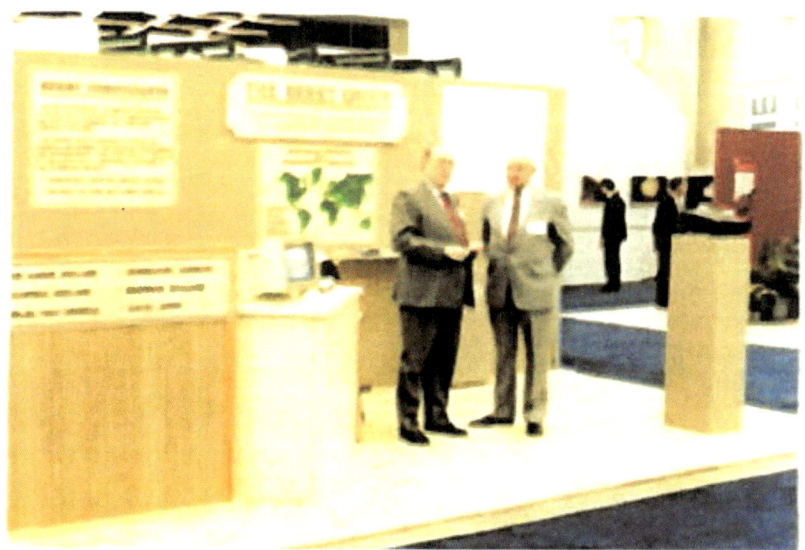

The BERKT exhibit at the Automotive Engineers Annual congress in
Detroit – 1990

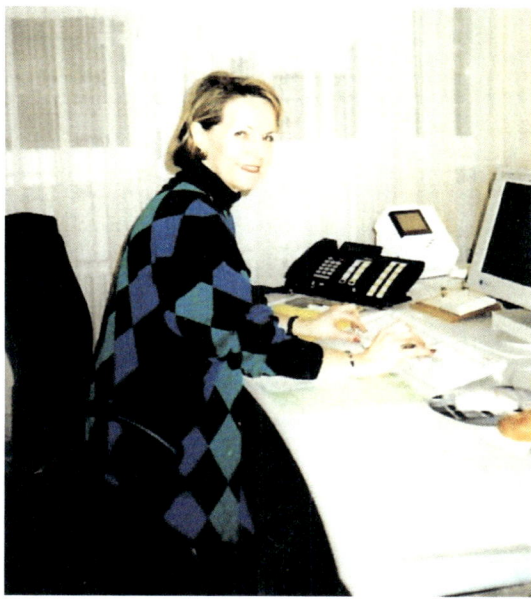

Anita in her office as associate director of wealth management –
Zurich 1990

Swiss politicians and some of the foreign notables living in nearby villas. It was always a memorable and happy occasion.

The sole male member at the party was myself as manservant for the Hens. I popped the champagne and wine, melted and scraped the cheese, and produced the crepes flambe. After the last bottle of wine was opened, all glasses were raised for the manservant's patience and good nature.

The decade of the eighties passed quickly, and Anita was promoted to Associate Director of the bank's wealth management department. I was managing a sixty-man group of consultants spread over offices in Zurich, Milan, Paris, Holland, England, Germany, and Michigan. The downside was not being able to spend enough time together at home with Anita.

The eighties were not all work and no fun—there was time for travel. Anita had six weeks' vacation and I could structure my work schedule to suit our plans.

In 1987 we made a much-awaited trip to Luxor in Egypt and spent ten days at the Swiss-run resort on Crocodile Island. Anita fell in love with the place at first sight.

"The place is beautiful, Parigi. We really lucked out. Our cabana is right next to the swimming pool and the dining room. And there's even a small zoo for the kids. I love it."

I was equally impressed and told her the place was managed by a Swiss couple and we shouldn't expect anything less than perfect

"The place looks great, Anita, but let's wait till after dinner for our judgment." As expected, the food was excellent.

We took a ferry across the Nile to visit tombs at the Valley of the Kings. A few weeks prior to our visit, a number of tourists there had been attacked and killed by terrorists, but Anita was not deterred. She had been studying hieroglyphics in Zurich and, as I expected, could read some of the inscriptions. She never ceased to impress me.

We cruised the museums at Luxor and Karnak, and made boat trips up and down the Nile with fellow tourists. She kept in touch for several years with some of those we had met.

The resort mascot was a large pelican named Cleo and was usually perched on a pole at the edge of the hotel swimming pool. When approached, Cleo would make gaggling sounds that intrigued Anita.

"Parigi, do you think she is speaking to us?"

My reply was predictable.

"Not in any language I recognize. She's probably begging for a fish handout, or maybe it's some forgotten Egyptian tongue you didn't

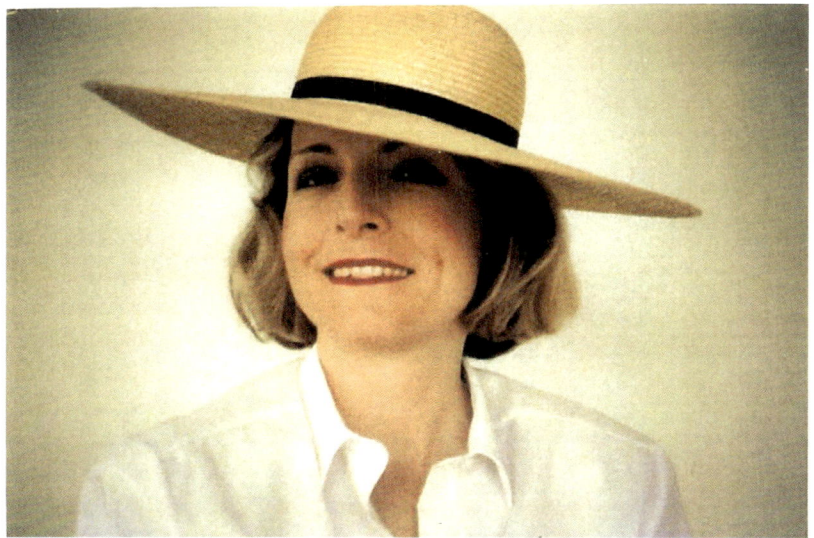

Anita drew more glances in Luxor than the ancient ruins.

come across in your hieroglyphs book. Let's go ask the old zookeeper if he speaks pelican."

"Parigi, you can never be serious. Birds certainly do communicate. She must be talking to us, because there is no other pelican around."

On the flight home, she insisted the pelican talked to us.

Having Anita alone with me for ten days on that island in the Nile was a memory never forgotten; one that often brought a bright smile to her face when I needed to see one.

We were joyfully in love and tuned our work schedules to focus on each others' personal needs. Every day away from her was a day lost—a day to be recovered through some gesture to her of my love and caring. The fact that I had turned sixty and Anita was forty-one played heavily on my mind and kept me focused on the challenges and opportunities of the coming decade. I knew there would be days of introspection, days when we would reflect on the wisdom and intent of the commitment we had made on that wonderful day in Las Vegas.

Chapter Four

SUNSHINE OF THE '90S

Anita and I worked hard through the next decade and were rewarded in both our careers. Anita continued to gain status in her banking position and BERKT continued to grow and achieve recognition and financial success in both Europe and America. The only downside was my having to spend half my time away from home.

Anita was being highly rewarded at the bank, but was unhappy about the salary discrimination suffered by other capable women colleagues. She spoke openly about her concern.

"Parigi, there are at least three other women at my level in the bank being paid twenty to twenty-five percent less than men doing the same work. I have to do something to shine a light on this, but I don't yet know how."

"I don't know what to tell you, Anita. I really doubt chauvinism can be completely eliminated in the business world, but in time, as more women move up the ladder, it might happen. The Swiss have always been notably chauvinistic, but I know that most women in my Scandinavian client companies and the Netherlands enjoy pay levels equal to men."

"I'm glad to hear that, hubby, because I'm starting an underground campaign with some influential women I know."

Her statement did not surprise me.

"Well, good for you. How are you going to bring about a change in your lifetime?"

"I'm not sure, but I'm hoping to use your status in the business world, and the help of some influential women in the business world who will participate."

"Okay, but only start something we can both agree on."

"Well, can we agree to entertain more often? Our reputation is good in that respect and we can host one or two educational dinner parties each month. I know several wives of owners and directors of the large Swiss companies I deal with at the bank and also know wives

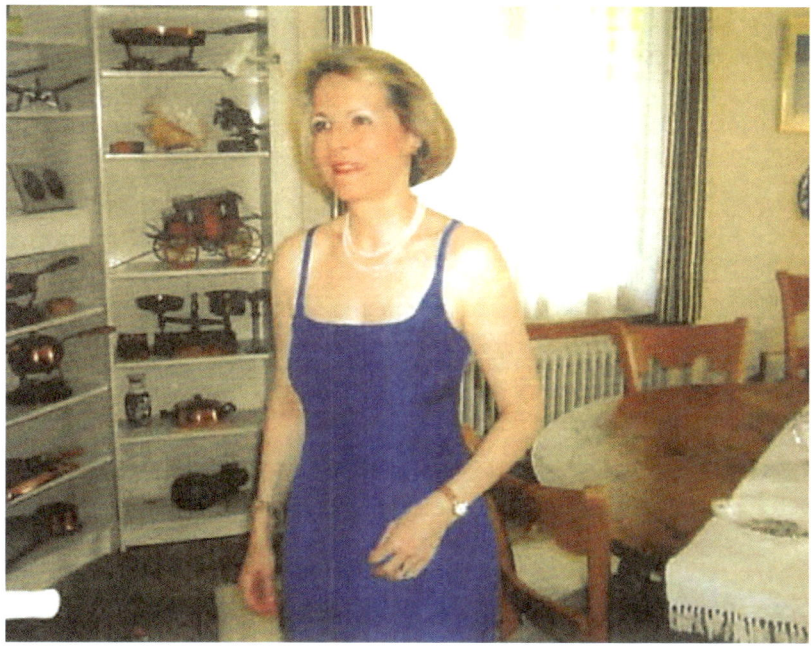

Anita – Always the beautiful hostess

of some big-shots at both the major and small private banks. It won't be difficult to get them to come here, and for some, if not all, to be brainwashed about women's equality."

"Remember, Anita, women didn't get to vote in canton Zurich until 1970, and it was 1971 before they could vote in the federal elections."

And that is how Anita's campaign for pay equality for women began. Her social influence in the community grew as well and she participated in town politics as a member of the dominant political party.

I was proud of her standing in the community and it was one of the reasons the village awarded me Swiss citizenship. My only concern was that too many of our friends and business associates wanted invitations to dinner—and I would have to do most of the cooking.

Anita turned fifty in October 1997, and I had promised her we would celebrate it in Paris for a week visiting our favorite hangouts and some of her Parisian friends.

She was radiant each day of our stay, and I saw the happiness in her eyes each morning at breakfast. She was so happy to be back in her favorite city, and I was happy just to be with her. It felt like we had never left our city of light for a less vibrant world, but our joyful interlude soon ended.

She looked back down the long station platform as we boarded the express train to Zurich and I saw her eyes moisten in a farewell that tugged at my heart.

By the end of the decade, there was a lot of attention being paid to women's equality throughout Europe and America. Anita's silent campaign in Zurich had begun to show some results. Women were slowly moving up the compensation ladder and Anita was encouraged.

"The end of the century is almost here, Parigi, and things will be getting better for women in the next decade, but nothing is certain, so we have to keep our campaign on track."

She was ever the optimist and I loved her for it.

While on a trip in 1992, to our office in Michigan, I had some chest pains and drove myself to the hospital. The doctor in the emergency room heard my story and thought I was nuts not to have called an ambulance. Next morning, I underwent placement of an artery stent.

Anita flew in from Zurich to provide the support I needed and got me back home. Three weeks later, I had chest pains and she took me to Hirslanden Hospital near our home where they discovered the first artery stent was improperly implanted. and the artery was again clogged. The stent was too short and a new one had to be inserted. Anita had the hospital send a letter to the Detroit cardiologist. There was no reply.

Anita was friendly with a wealthy and influential patroness of the hospital for children in Zurich. Because of this friendship, Anita and I attended several fundraising dinners each year and made frequent visits to the hospital to bring small gifts and some cheer to the children. It was a labor of love for both of us and often brought tears when we departed.

I had brought up the subject of children with Anita and each time her reply was the same.

"Parigi, it wouldn't have been fair for a child to be cared for by a nanny most of the time. Our careers demand too much time, and that doesn't count the time spent on necessary social and community affairs. Anyway, once I turned thirty-five, I realized it was too late for us to bring a child into this world."

My answer was always the same.

"It's not too late for us to adopt. I don't want you to be without a child of your own to be with you in your later years. My kids and

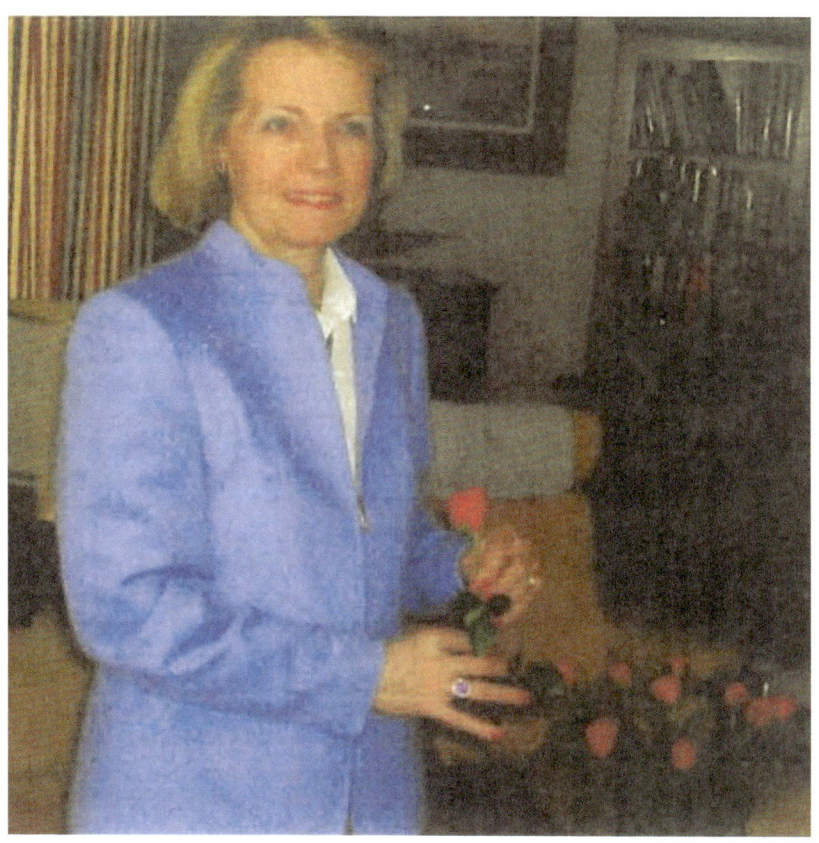

Anita after her 45th birthday dinner – 1992
The roses were also beautiful.

grandkids love you, but it's not the same. It leaves me with a deep feeling of guilt when I think of you being alone should something happen to me."

I saw the love and affection she had for the children at the hospital, and saw the regret in her eyes each time we left them. I saw sadness in her eyes at Christmas as we went through the ritual of trimming our tree at the window overlooking the lake. I could read it in her face—a child was missing.

Her sister once told her: "When I drive home from the city each night, I look up to your place on the hillside. I see your tree winking out the window at me and I feel good."

During the rest of the '90s, we were deeply involved in our careers and socially involved in our community. Anita had a wide range of friends, including Lillian, a Chinese woman, who owned a chain of high-end boutiques in Singapore, Hong Kong, and Canada. Lillian made buying trips to Paris, Zurich, and Milan twice a year and often stopped over in Zurich. She was always a welcome guest in our home.

Lillian and Anita talked fashion and discussed Anita's clothing designs from her couture studio days in the seventies when we lived in Paris. Lillian urged her to come up with a line of skirts and slacks that could be promoted in her boutiques in Asia.

"Parigi, it was difficult to turn down her offer, even though it would have been a new adventure."

We roamed Europe on our vacation during the better part of the decade. Paris was always on our agenda and we added Holland and the Scandinavian countries as well. Anita was always upbeat, never too tired to travel, and always well read before we left for a new destination. Milan, Italy was a two-hour drive from Zurich and we went there to see friends almost every month. We often discussed the prospect of moving there when we retired.

We closed out the decade in good health and anticipation for the new century on our doorstep. Anita remained socially active in the community and persistent in her fitness program. I knew she would outlast me.

Chapter Five

A DECADE OF CHANGE

We opened the new century in Fall River, Massachusetts by hosting a party in the Captains Club overlooking Battleship Bay. We brought Marie van Dyke, the widow of an old BERKT colleague who had been the Prima Soprano of the Dutch National Opera. Marie had agreed to sing for the group, but the pianist my cousin had hired failed to show up and Anita was very embarrassed. A little of the occasion was saved when we played one of her arias from a music disc, I had thought to bring with me.

Anita was stunning in her evening gown and, as was her way, spent time with each and every guest. In turn, I was deluged by questions about my beautiful and gracious wife and her home in the Swiss Alps. One question was answered more than once.

"No, she did not milk goats and no, she did not make Swiss cheese."

She had only one complaint about the party.

"I wish you had not given those smelly cigars to every man in the room."

As usual, she was the center of attraction that night. The men in attendance ranged in age from sixteen to eighty-six, and a few of the women smirked as she danced with each one.

Anita arranged another millennium party in Zurich. This time it was in the restaurant owned by her brother, Thomas. Most of our friends and all her family members attended. The food, wine, ambiance, and service were excellent. Her smile and happiness were contagious from each welcome to the ciao at each departure. It was a special occasion that remained a subject of discussion for many months and the memory of her beauty on that night will remain with me forever.

Unlike the slight anxiety she showed at the Fall River party, she remained relaxed and content at her brother Tommy's place, from beginning to end.

"This was a wonderful party, Parigi. My feet were not tromped on once—unlike the abuse they took in Fall River. Best of all, there was no choking cigar smoke and this time the food was excellent. Remember how, in Fall River, the food quality had been a roll of the dice?"

The first decade of the new century produced career challenges for both Anita and myself.

An economic downturn in both America and Europe had deeply reduced budgets for the hiring of consultants. By 2002, contracting of consultants by both carmakers and component manufacturers had been reduced by half that of the previous decade.

I was concerned by the aging of my colleagues. Two of whom had recently been lost to debilitating illnesses and their knowledge and experience would be difficult to replace.

Anita kept abreast of business conditions and was supportive when we sat and discussed our future prospects.

"Remember, Parigi, you have been very successful for more than twenty years. Now you're twenty years older and deserve a chance to slow down and spend more time with me at home."

She was right, of course. I could afford to slow down.

Her own career at the bank was uncertain due to a merger with another large Swiss bank, but there was a chance of her taking early retirement under very favorable conditions.

"You're right, Anita. Maybe now is the time for us to slow down a bit. We have no financial worries, and I really would like to spend more time on my writing and painting—I still haven't painted your portrait."

As predicted, Anita and several other key managers at the bank were given the opportunity for early retirement at full pension in 2004. Her going away party was somewhat sad for she was leaving behind a successful, twenty-four-year banking career, and losing her day-to-day interface with longtime colleagues, but she soon settled into her new lifestyle and became more involved in local politics, charity work for children, and action on behalf of equal rights for women.

We had time to travel and took the opportunity to visit our favorite places in Italy, France, Spain, Austria, and every inch of Switzerland. We visited Manhattan—a place of so many memories for Anita and saw the Christmas show at Radio City Music Hall and two Broadway musicals.

When members of my family came to visit, Anita had an open and loving embrace to all. She doted on my grandchildren and each one responded with tenderness and love.

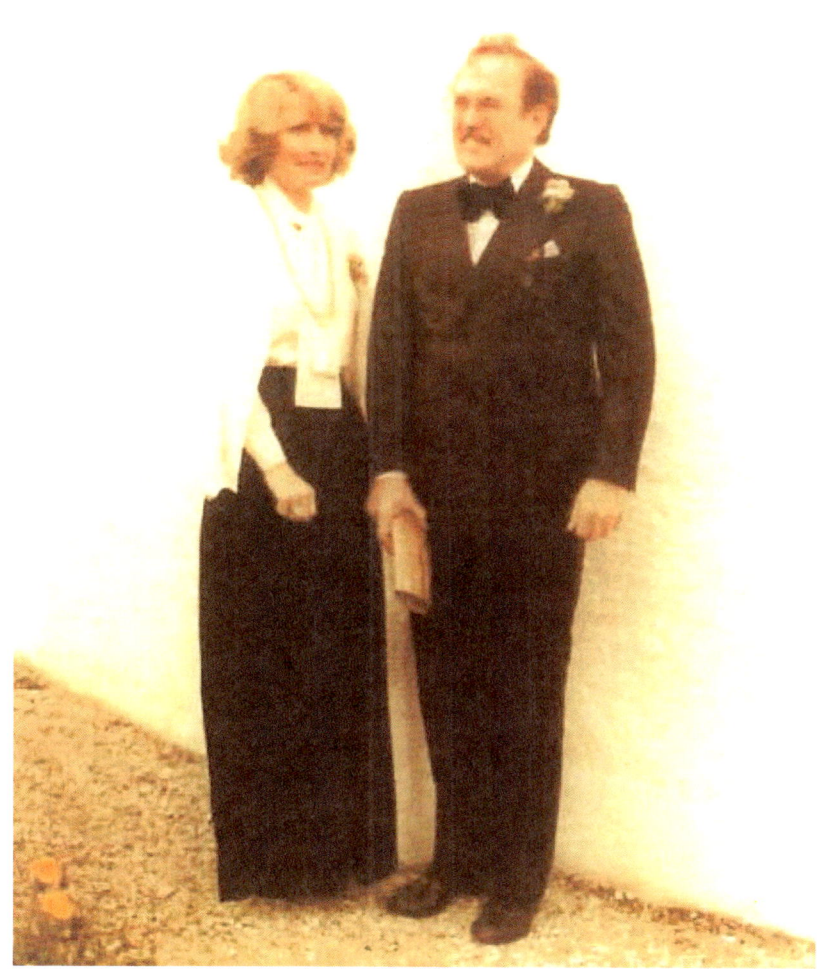

Waiting for the wedding to start 2006

In April, 2006, Anita's friend, whose father owned a private bank in Zurich, announced her coming marriage and insisted we attend. Her father had reserved a hotel on a lake for the three-day occasion, and when we arrived at our suite, Anita was overwhelmed.

"My God, Parigi, this is one of the finest suites in the hotel. I know she is a good friend, but I hadn't expected such grand treatment. I know her papa owns a bank, but he has the reputation of being a skinflint."

There was no truth to her statement. Anita deserved all that came her way. She was always grateful and never failed to acknowledge any gift, favor, love, or kindness, and was always a little guilty when she felt she received more than she deserved.

During our many trips through the western states, she had become aware of the needs of American Indian children and was a regular donor to several Indian schools and often felt her annual donations were not enough.

The wedding eve dinner was complete with a ten-piece dance band playing modern swing—appropriate for the setting and the average age of the guests. Anita hummed the tunes as we danced and received nods and smiles from couples on the floor. When the music went up-tempo, we chose to sit it out to sip wine on a sofa by the windows overlooking the moonlit lake.

We were fervent music lovers and over the years Anita became a fan of American country and western music and hits from the big-band era. I had a pretty good singing voice, and on long road trips, I would sing to pass the time. She usually fell asleep. Maybe it was to drown out my voice.

On the wedding day, we boarded a paddle-wheel lake steamer, but the wedding couple were not on board. We were told the couple would board at the next village after attending to some formalities.

A six-tiered wedding cake sat on the main table of the twenty-table dining salon and drew a comment from Anita.

"My father had wanted a big affair for our wedding, Parigi, but nothing as spectacular as this."

"Anita, your father doesn't own a bank."

That evening every place in the dining room had a personal thank-you card from the bride and groom. At each table was a bucket with three bottles of the finest French champagne, at end of evening, all were empty. On our drive home, I confessed my feelings about the whole affair.

"I couldn't stop thinking of how much you deserved the same treatment. You deserved much more than the little chapel in Las Vegas and more than a wedding suite at Caesars Palace. Thinking about what you missed, leaves me with an empty feeling of guilt."

"Oh, Parigi! You know you will always be my loving hubby—even though you snore sometimes."

Over the next four years, we made trips around Europe, America, Africa, and Asia. Each summer we vacationed in our favorite seaside towns in Italy—Senegal on the Adriatic and Forte dei Marmi on the Mediterranean. We had many friends in Italy who welcomed us with open arms, and seeing them brought us both great joy.

In April, 2008, Anita said she had never been to Morocco.

"Parigi, some friends at the fitness club told me about a dream hotel in Agadir where the rooms are only seventy Swiss Francs a night. It's on the beach and the rooms and food are excellent. Maybe we can look into it for our next trip."

I was open and recalled a trip I made to Agadir in earlier years.

"Agadir has some small shops that custom-make leather jackets. They are beautifully made and cost about one quarter of what you would pay in Zurich. You'll go nuts when you see some of that leather stuff."

The flight was two hours, and on the approach, we flew over thousands of hot houses growing flowers for European markets.

I made an observation for Anita.

"Half those places down there are growing pot."

"Oh, Parigi, why do you provide such unnecessary information?"

"I don't know, sweety. I guess I remember too much. That's always been one of my weaknesses."

She jabbed my arm and narrowed her eyes.

"There you go again. Why can't you be serious?"

We thoroughly enjoyed our vacation, and Anita flew home with one red and one pink leather jacket for little more than two hundred Swiss Francs.

In October of that year, we visited one of Anita's old bank colleagues in Tokyo and I introduced her to the Kabuki theater and my favorite sushi bar on the Ginza. We stayed at the Palace Hotel and, though she was skittish about taking off her clothes in front of other residents, we enjoyed the hotel's luxurious public bath and the meticulous attention paid her by the girl pool attendants.

In later years, her memory of it was sharp.

"I would never do that again. Once was an adventure—twice would be obscene indulgence."

I arranged a stopover in Hong Kong and another in Bangkok on our way back from Tokyo. We had a suite in the Regent Hotel in Hong Kong overlooking the harbor and sat at the window for tea to watch the ferries, ships, and local junks plying the Kowloon channel below in a seemingly endless line.

One of my former clients was a wealthy Hong Kong businessman who owned an electric components company. His wife had been educated in Switzerland and took to Anita right away. Together they toured the city in her limousine, shopped, and had tea in the Peninsular Hotel. Anita was impressed with her new friend's bargaining ability.

"Parigi, she never paid the asking price for anything. She would get what she wanted for much less than the shop was asking."

In Bangkok we stayed at the Oriental Hotel, across the river from the royal palace and the emerald pagoda. One night we were entertained by traditional Thai dancers at a place near the pagoda. Anita talked about it often and I was happy she had seen a few more beautiful sights from my earlier life.

The Oriental Hotel laid on a grand lunch every noon on their riverside terrace. The main foot tables stretched thirty feet, and the dessert and fruit table—ten. The main items were Thai, but included Japanese, Chinese, English, and French selections. All were excellent and it was almost sinful not to overindulge.

Anita was overwhelmed. "Parigi, I've never seen such a spread. The buffets in Sweden were tiny, compared to this. Tell me you didn't eat here every day when you lived in Bangkok."

"No, not really. Only on Sundays."

Anita bought two paintings by a well-known Thai artist and hung them on our dining room wall for our dinner guests to admire. She always pointed out her husband's paintings hanging nearby.

Home in Zurich, our daily routine did not change much. On weekends we walked in the mountain valleys and along the shores of Lake Zurich, did fitness training, attended the opera, and concerts at the famous Tonhalle. We were active in village politics and busy raising money for the children's hospital. Our circle of friends grew and we were kept on dinner lists year around. We were active and content.

Chapter Six

LAST YEARS IN ZURICH

On one night in May of 2010, while I was busy completing one of the wooden ship models in my collection, I heard a cry for help from Anita. I rushed to the bathroom and found her on the floor in a pool of blood.

She was conscious and struggling to sit up.

"What happened? Did you trip on something?"

I reached for a towel to stop the blood streaming from a gash on her head and raised her to her feet.

"No. I just blacked out when I was taking off my makeup. I guess I fell against the tub. It hurts!"

I got her dressed and drove to the emergency room at Hirslanden Hospital where her wound was stitched and I was told there was no sign of a concussion. I was to keep her in bed for a day and watch to be sure she was staying alert and was able to walk steadily.

To my great relief, a thorough examination a week later showed nothing that could account for her blackout.

In June and July of 2010, we made trips to our favorite spots in Italy—Forte dei Marmi, Desenzano, Senigallia, and Venice were alive and welcoming. We soaked up the sun, the sea breeze, our favorite wines, and foods at our old hangouts. On our last night, it struck me that this might be our last visit. It proved to be true.

In August, after roaming the annual village fair with some of our neighbors, we had dinner at a local, eighteenth-century inn in the village. I broached a subject we had discussed a few weeks earlier.

"We have often talked about some potential retirement sites we've visited. Should we talk about that some more?"

She looked down at her plate for a few seconds.

"Yes, Parigi, it's been on my mind also. I guess we should talk. If I said we should move to Italy, I know you would not object, but that would not be my choice. I think we should be somewhere closer to your family. And when you are gone, I can return to Zurich. I want to spend my last days here where we first met and were happy for so many years."

"Anita, I promise that wherever we wind up, we will spend a holiday here each year and wherever else you wish to go."

"Thank you, Parigi. We do have to maintain ties with our home ground and must never forget our life here. I did like some of the places we looked at on the Connecticut shore and some places we looked at near your friends in North Carolina, but I think we should set up a temporary base in New England until we make the final decision on a location."

I agreed and told her we would be financially secure with our pensions, savings, and our investment portfolios. I assured her our monthly income would go further in America than it would in Zurich

"Remember, we always have the option of coming back here if you are not happy with our life in America."

"Let's try to make a good life in America, Parigi. We both have friends there. You have children and grandchildren to visit you, and I always enjoyed going to your oldest daughter's place in Vermont for Thanksgiving. I loved sitting in front of the fireplace with your grandchildren and their little ones. I look forward to doing that again."

In July of 2011, our household goods were shipped to America. Anita handled all the details with a shipping company she had worked with in New York City. She closed our local bank accounts and informed the town office of our move.

When the movers had departed, we stood alone in the home we had loved for twenty-eight years. We stood, hand-in hand at the living room window where the Christmas tree was decorated each year to gaze one last time to the green hills across the lake. I pointed to the ridge path we had walked so many Sundays.

Anita's grip on my hand tightened and there was slight resistance as we turned away from the window. I saw the tears. I kissed and caressed her as we went down the two flights of stairs to the street. We walked down the hill to the railroad station platform and boarded a train to the airport and our flight to Boston.

Anita's sisters, her brother, and three of her old bank colleagues were waiting in the airport hotel lobby. I knew the last lunch we had planned would be a sad occasion for her and did my best to keep the conversations upbeat.

As we sat with our friends for that last lunch, my mind took a detour to an earlier lunch with my friend and lawyer, Alfred. We were

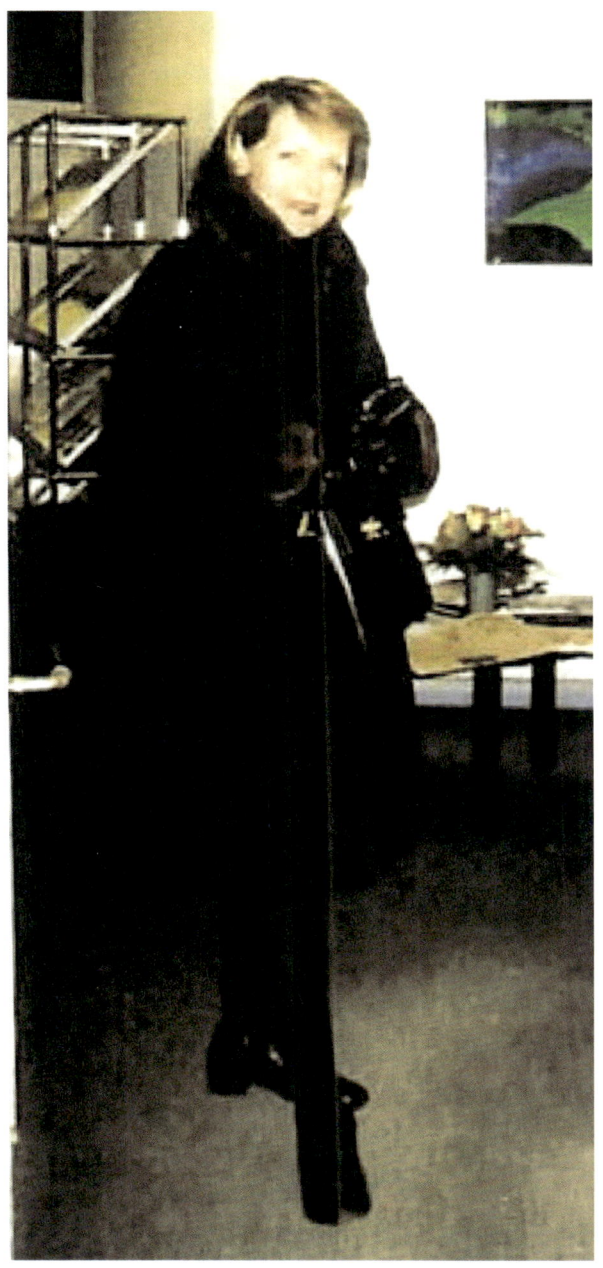

2012 - Concert night

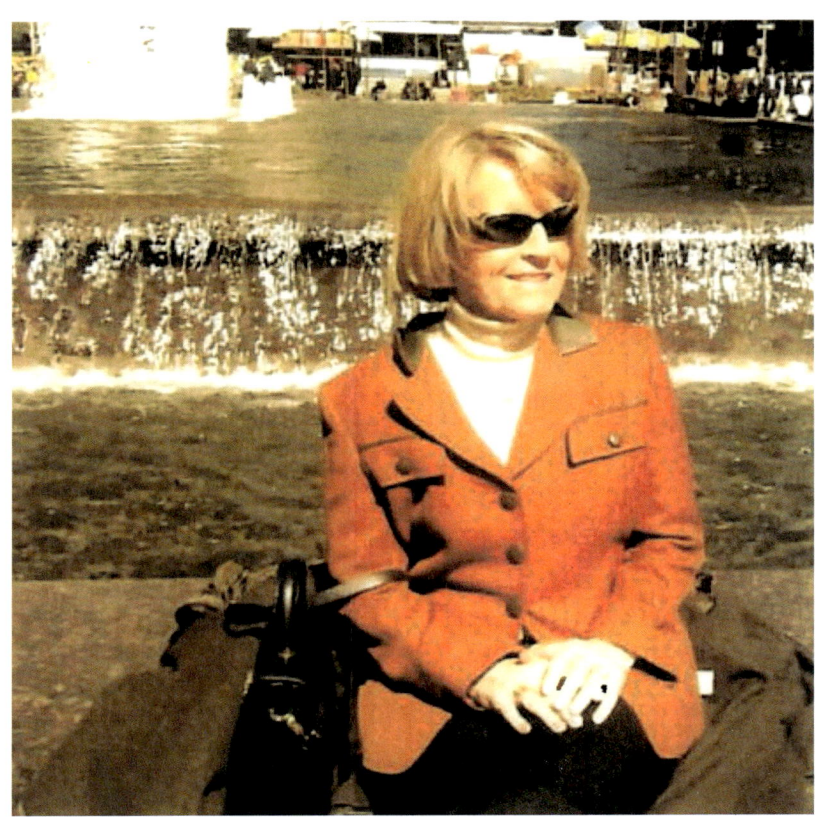

Anita's last day in Manhattan (March 2012)

having our usual Thursday lunch of steamed mussels when I announced the decision to move to America.

"Al, there are so many things we can do together. If I had my way, I'd buy another boat and spend summers cruising out of Bristol and up the coast to Martha's Vineyard, Nantucket, and Kennebunk, Maine. I had a home at Kennebunk Beach for a couple of years."

Al squinted. "Sounds like a plan, my friend. While you are playing Captain Ahab chasing Moby Dick, how will Anita occupy herself? You know she's not a sailor; she didn't like boating, even on placid lake Zurich"

"Oh, we'll make plenty of road trips and she'll enjoy more of America's wonders. She often says America is a great and beautiful land deserving more of our attention."

Al was skeptical. He wondered why Anita would drive thousands of miles to satisfy her husband's wanderlust. The conversation would come back to haunt me later.

"She's right, Anita. You do have what it takes, but I will tell her you have been a star since the day you were born."

Back in Rhode Island, we found a temporary apartment not far from where I grew up and only a thirty-minute drive from the seashore. There was a local college nearby with a winter concert schedule and we enjoyed attending twice a month.

Most of February, 2012 was consumed by steps taken to obtain Anita's resident green card, which was granted in March.

We went to Manhattan in March and met with our portfolio manager to make some investment adjustments. Anita was in high spirits and shopped at Sax Fifth Avenue while I went to Brooks Brothers for some of my needs.

"We have to come down more often, Parigi. I have fond memories of my six years working here."

I agreed, not knowing it would be an unkept promise.

Chapter Seven

EARLY SIGNS OF A PROBLEM

In May of 2012, Anita agreed to make a trip to visit my son Brad and his family in Michigan. She had become close to Brad, his wife and two boys, so I thought it would be a pleasant visit.

Brad's place was a ten-hour drive away and for the first time, Anita declined to help with the driving. She showed signs of distraction and it troubled me. She was usually very attentive and questioned me about places along the route.

She was not her usual outgoing self during our visit and seemed reluctant to converse with those who were not a part of the family. On the third day, she told me she was anxious to get back home and go to the beach.

I offered my apologies and said Anita was not feeling well and it was best that we headed home. Anita invited them all to come to Rhode Island during the summer vacation to spend some time with us on the Atlantic seashore.

Anita slept for most of the drive home and when we stopped for food, I asked if she was not feeling well.

"I'm fine, Parigi. Don't worry."

I was not convinced and pressed her.

"Did something at Brad's place upset you?"

She looked down at her lap and sighed.

"No. I'm just tired from the trip. I'll be happy to sleep in our own bed once again. Our bed at Brad's place was very uncomfortable."

By the time we arrived home, she was relaxed and her usual outgoing and chatty self. By October we had settled into a morning routine of fitness and lunch at one of the small places we liked. One was a small golf club where Anita enjoyed a view of the fairway from her favorite seat at the bar. She talked to the bar maids and members of the club and took interest in golf.

"Parigi, maybe you could teach me to play before it snows, or do you think that's too optimistic?"

"You learn fast, Anita, but it would be better to start your training at the golf driving range."

We made a few trips to the driving range before she decided golf was not to be her game.

Rhode Island College was only ten minutes away and I bought two season tickets for the 2012 winter concerts and dance performances. Anita enjoyed shows that were lively and rhythmic—things like the TAO drummers and the South African dancers. On two occasions, when the concerts were somewhat somber, she wanted to go home at intermission and watch one of her favorite TV shows. Although I was enjoying the concerts, I did not insist that we stay. I cannot remember her having done that at any of the many concerts we attended in Europe, and I was concerned.

Each weekday morning Anita put on her gym clothes and led me out the door to the fitness club. She was admired and welcomed at the club and used most of the exercise machines available. I couldn't understand why she showed no sweat or fatigue after working out for two hours. In my case, workouts were limited to the treadmill, bicycle, leg-push machines, bar bell lifts, and a hot shower when finished.

On weekends, weather permitting, we drove to Bristol and walked the bay shore path at Colt State Park for two hours before going to Aiden's Pub for lunch. Anita enjoyed the quaint pub and the trio of Irish musicians that entertained each weekend. In winter, real logs burned in the brick fireplace. The waitresses were friendly and efficient, the atmosphere was always pleasant and the prices reasonable. Anita always ordered blueberry or the strawberry-rhubarb pie for dessert.

She never tired of our road trips and was more relaxed in the car than sitting at home. She enjoyed walking and we spent hours in local parks and at the rocky shores of Narragansett and Newport.

She was always a history buff and enjoyed our trips to Boston, eager to learn its history. I introduced her to Quincy Market and many of the famous eating places, including the Union Oyster House, the oldest continuously operating eating house in America. Several times we sat at the famous oyster bar and downed a platter of little-necks on the half-shell and a glass of white wine while I told her of famous people who had sat at the bar in generations past.

During the Thanksgiving period, we visited my cousins in the area. On those occasions Anita was withdrawn and showed signs of anxiety when we spent more than an hour. During a visit with my brother, she remained silent and unwilling to join in conversation. She liked my brother, so this sudden change was troubling.

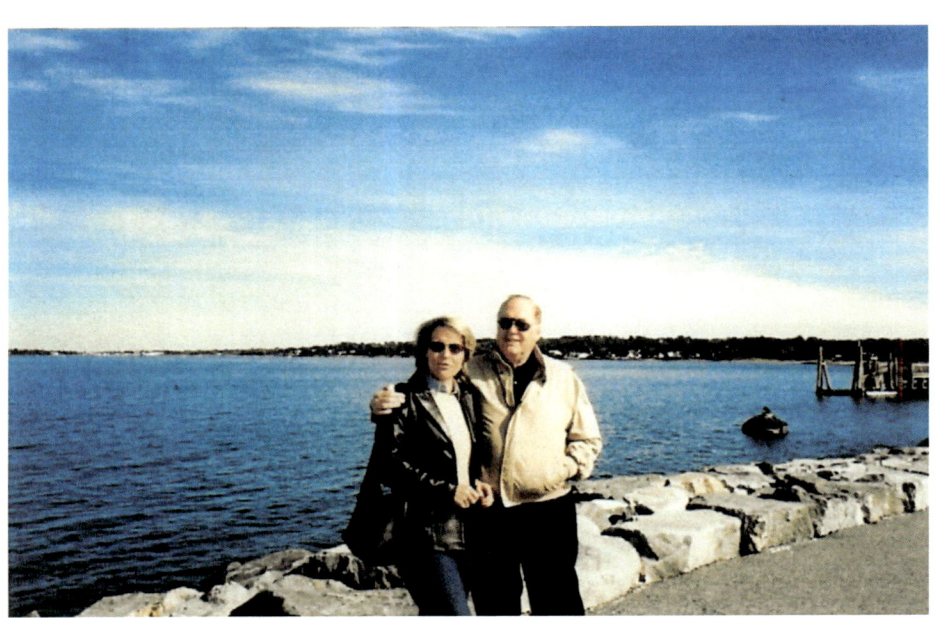

A Sunday walk at Colt State Park (2012)

I became more concerned when she had trouble identifying items in the refrigerator, and sometimes she would stand looking at her coffee machine until I asked if something was wrong.

"Yes. I can't find the filter. It was right here yesterday. Did you take it?"

"No, sweety. It's right here next to the coffee can."

This didn't happen every day, but often enough to worry me, so I made an appointment with a neurologist. I was given a prescription for anxiety pills and told some memory loss in a woman of sixty was not unusual. If her condition worsened, I was to bring her back for further examination.

A prescription for anti-anxiety pills was given with advice to keep her active and calm.

"Well, Doc, how in hell do I keep her active and calm at the same time?"

"Have her do something she likes to do outside the house. If her memory fail much more, we can do a scan to see what's going on."

This limited advice prompted me to do some research on the complications of dementia in otherwise fit and athletic women. I soon learned that memory loss was not a subject of major research in the American health system.

Christmas that year was the second time a natural tree was not sitting in our living room—apartment house rules permitted only synthetic trees. Anita was depressed until I found an easily assembled tree with lights. When she saw it, her mood lightened and she spent the evening decorating the tree with ornaments we had remembered to bring from Zurich.

I was concerned when she could not recall the origin of most of the decorations—she had always remembered the date and origin of each one. On reflection, I had also forgotten the details.

We decided to drive to Vermont and spend Christmas with my daughter, her six children, and five grandchildren. Anita was relaxed and as we drove; we discussed the motel where we would stay in Woodstock.

"There are not enough beds at the farm. So, we'll stay in the Shire Motel. You remember the Shire. It's the place you liked so much last time."

She smiled and nodded.

"Yes, and I love that quaint café where we have breakfast. Woodstock is the most beautiful town in Vermont."

"It certainly is, and remember that my grandson Ben has a new baby girl for you to cuddle."

"You didn't tell me about that. What's her name and how old is she?"

I said he name was Nora. "She is two months old and you'll love her."

When we arrived at the farm she saw Nora, and asked to hold her. She cuddled and kissed her little nose and hands for over an hour and was disappointed when she gave her up for a feeding. In her eyes I saw the regret for her not having a child of her own. In turn, I felt the guilt of not making more of an effort to change her mind about having at least one child of our own. It remains with me forever.

Back in Rhode Island, we greeted the new year cuddled on our sofa in front of our wide-screen television and watched the traditional Vienna State Orchestra perform their annual concert, but deep in our minds we were home in Zurich watching the concert. I had even more doubt about my taking this beautiful woman from her home in Switzerland.

We take a holiday in the Bahamas

In March of 2013, I arranged a trip to Nassau in the Bahamas. Anita had told me she wanted to visit the islands and see if they were all they're advertised to be. She was calm and relaxed on the flight from Orlando, but when we landed in Nassau, she became animated.

"Parigi, I could see the beach hotels when we came in for the landing. Our hotel must have been down there. What was the hotel name again?"

Her question surprised me. She had chosen the hotel from the travel brochure and told our neighbors about it several times.

"Oh, come now. You remember. We're at Sunset Beach. The one with the casino and indoor pool."

She tilted her head and gave me a sweet grin.

"I remember now. I like a swimming pool. The ocean is full of sharks and jellyfish."

"Don't worry. The only critters in the pool will have two legs."

It took me several minutes to get checked in while Anita sat in the lounge, sipped iced tea, and watched several small children giggle as they ran around her chair. She was already enjoying herself.

Each morning we dug into the breakfast buffet and Anita loaded her plate with fresh fruit, egg salad and a fresh bagel. We sat at a window table to eat and read a copy of a German newspaper from the hotel bookstore.

"Parigi, I would like to read the *Neue Zürcher Zeitung* and learn about what's going on back home."

"I thought about it, Anita. When we get home, I'll order a weekly copy from a paper store I know in New York City."

She smiled and asked the expected question.

"When will we be able to go back home again?"

I thought she meant going back to Zurich for a visit, but I wasn't sure.

"If you like, we can plan a visit for this September. It would be better to and be there after the summer tourists are gone and before it snows in Pontresina."

Anita stayed off the beach sand, wouldn't wade in the water, and refused to sit at the beach bar for a drink. She preferred sitting by the hotel pool watching the children play. It was disturbing to see her become much less communicative as we approached the end of our visit.

We made a tour of the shopping area in the city and she found a beautiful tanzanite and diamond ring in a small jewelry shop. I haggled with the shop owner, reached a satisfactory price, and slipped the ring on her finger.

"You deserve this. It's been a long time since I gave my lovely wife something almost as beautiful as herself."

She gazed at her finger every few minutes most of our remaining time in Nassau.

On our next to last day, I fell and bruised my ribs. The hotel nurse taped me up, but my chest was sore for a week. Anita was anxious, but I assured her.

"Don't worry, this clumsy clunker can still sail when the wind is astern."

She smiled, patted my arm and I wondered if she still remembered our sailing days on Narragansett Bay. She was always anxious when aboard my sloop, but went along to please me and gradually learned the terms of the sport.

There was an incident on the flight home from Orlando that upset me.

Contrary to her gentle way with children, Anita slapped the hand of a small boy in the seat behind her. He had repeatedly reached between the seat to pull Anita's hair. The mother sat across the aisle and stood to admonish Anita until the flight attendant arrived.

I was furious and explained what the boy had been doing, but she said I should have called her to confront the boy's mother. Anita sat in silence for the rest of the flight and the taxi ride home. From that point on, she rarely talked to anyone but me. When someone addressed her, she uttered a few words in reply, and spoke to me only in Swiss-German or French. It was disturbing and I was at a loss for what to do.

Our primary physician said Anita was showing early signs of dementia, but was otherwise healthy. I didn't believe him.

We continued our regular routine of fitness club visits, and on most days, we had lunch at one of the local taverns. Anita had become accustomed to the waitresses and regular customers at each place and rarely strayed from her usual food choices of fish and chips, calamari, or half a sandwich with a cup of soup. A year earlier her food selections had been wider and more tasty.

We drove to Vermont for Thanksgiving so Anita could be again with my great-granddaughter, Nora. Once there, she was more alert, smiled a lot and interacted with each of the older children, but spent most of her time in front of the fireplace with Nora on her lap. She was content and happy during the time we spent at the farm and the only sadness she showed was during her farewell kiss to Nora and each of the older children.

I set up our tree on the first week of December, just as we had dome in Switzerland. Anita helped with the decorating and smiled happily when I switched on the red, green, and blue tree lights. When it was done, we cuddled on the sofa. The tree winked and we watched Anita's favorite TV series, *Gunsmoke*.

PART IV

Chapter Eight

TIME TO START A DIARY

During November and December of 2013, Anita had occasional night-time coughing spells. They became more frequent over the following two months, so in December, I took her to a woman oncologist. An x-ray revealed a small spot on her lung. I was told it was in a precarious position and taking a biopsy would be dangerous—she would have to be monitored every two months for any changes. I was deeply concerned and decided to keep a periodic record of her condition.

January 10th, 2014: Met with the oncologist and she ordered blood work and scheduled a C-scan for Anita.

January 14th: Took Anita for blood work, but she refused to submit and the nurse gave up. I don't know why a blood sample is needed for a C-scan.

January 17th: Anita drank the barium given to her by the oncology nurse and went to the hospital only to learn the oncologist had cancelled the procedure without notifying me. I was furious.

January 18th: Anita went to the kitchen while I was asleep and put a plastic food container on the stove. I smelled something burning, jumped out of bed, and was able to remove the container before the smoke alarm went off. I removed all the stove control knobs. With each passing day, I become more worried about my lovely wife. I cannot bare to think of what life would be without her.

January 20th: I visited the local Alzheimer's center for information and guidance. The staff members were friendly and provided a paper describing the. Seven stages. I have done some research on my own about the progression of this insidious ailment and learned little from the visit.

I will make every effort or stop her decline and have been told there will be more bad than good days, but I will fill her life with the love and care she deserves, no matter what it takes.

January 27th: Took Anita to lunch at the tavern and she had a few words with the regulars. We watched TV at home for an hour and she fell asleep until 7:00 p.m. I got her to remove her makeup, brush her teeth, and put on her nightgown. She was in bed by 8:00 p.m. She smiled during the process but didn't say a word. I chalked it up to fatigue.

January 28th: Anita was out of bed at 4:00 a.m. and lay on the living room couch for three hours in her dress slacks and a blouse. She resisted when I made her change into her fitness outfit—she said she wanted to look good when we went to the coffee shop. Her workout was mostly treadmill, bicycle, and ten-pound weight lifts. She is always enthusiastic and is able to keep pace with me.

We went home for lunch, but when she saw the stove controls missing, she headed for the door. I had to chase her down the hall twice, before she would settle down and eat her lunch.

I sat with her all afternoon and thumbed through our photo albums. She had difficulty naming people in the photos that we had known for many years. It depressed me.

January 30th: Mollie, a part-time caregiver, came in at noon and took Anita for a two-hour walk in Lincoln Park, and once back home, Mollie trimmed and polished Anita's fingernails. I haven't seen her so calm and relaxed for several weeks. I hope it's a sign of better days to come.

I continued research on Alzheimer's disease and was discouraged by how little I found beyond papers on the stages of progression, amyloid buildup on the brain. Statistics available on the growing number of cases in the population were very discouraging.

Discussions with our primary physician only confirmed how little help I could expect in the coming months.

"Paris, all we can do is monitor her condition and try some medications that may slow her decline"

He was confirming only what I already knew.

"Yes, Doc, I know there are areas in medicine where treatment is still a black art."

He smiled, shrugged, and nodded. I took it to be reluctant agreement. The AMA would have been unhappy about his confession.

February 5th: It has been a tough winter with snow and cold for the past six weeks. Anita sits and watches me cook, bake, and do laundry or sits on her easy chair to look out on the balcony and watch the birds peck at the seed she puts out daily. Her favorites are two gray turtle doves, a cardinal, and two bluebirds. She waves her hands to admonish them when they bully the smaller wrens and sparrows.

February 10th: Anita fell off the treadmill at the fitness club and hurt her knee. A sports physician club member was able to examine her and said it was just a bad bruise. I brought her home and applied an icepack and there was only slight swelling. I will take her for an x-ray tomorrow as a caution.

February 20th: I had to put a security cap on the door to keep Anita from wandering out of the apartment without me. Somehow, she removed the cap and walked around the building while I was cooking. I know she is in the "Sundowner Stage," and will have to watch her every minute from here on.

I gave her an anti-anxiety pill and we drove to Bristol for lunch at Aiden's Pub. She is always at ease there. We sat by the cozy fireplace and, as always, she had her favorite—fish and chips and her glass of Stella beer. The meal was topped off with our favorite—a dish of hot blueberry pie a la mode. She was smiling and relaxed on the drive home

February 22nd: Mollie watched Anita while I went to Massachusetts to visit my cousin Beverly. I said I have been depressed for days and explained why. "It was a big mistake to take Anita from Switzerland—a big mistake—one I will rue for the rest of my life."

Beverly tried to console me by describing the pain she had endured while her father and mother had lived with her. My uncle had come down with Alzheimer's and passed away in her home when he was seventy-three. Her description of his last years was the opposite of consoling.

"Beverly, Anita is only sixty-three. She deserves many more years with me at her side. It was wrong to take her away from her home. She sacrificed herself for me. I don't know how to make it up to her and I weep over what I have done to her life. I know I must endure months of anguish, but she will get all the love and care I can give, no matter what the cost or effort."

March 4th: Below freezing today. We went to fitness club and stopped at Dunkin Donuts for coffee and Anita's bagel with cream cheese.

She set the table for dinner, but forgot some items. After the meal she stood holding her coat until I took her out to see a Brazilian dance troupe perform at Rhode Island College. She responds well to music and dancing and the show might have reminded her of our nights in Sao Paulo where samba groups flooded the streets and marched through the restaurants while we were eating. She was very happy there and always gave a tip to the dancers.

Anita enjoyed every minute the Brazilians were on stage, but when the final curtain came down, she stood and said, "Oh no," with a sad smile of disappointment. I have to take her out to more performances because music and dance are good forms of therapy. I sing her favorite songs when we're driving somewhere, but it's not the same as a stage performance.

March 12th: Woke up this morning with Anita standing at bedside with her coat and hat in hand. In the kitchen I saw she made coffee with the Italian expresso machine and it was good to see her doing something for herself. On the other hand, she gets confused when I ask her to bring me something from the kitchen—she often brings the wrong thing.

After I coaxed her into a warm water shower to relaxed her, we left for the fitness club. She has put on weight and I had a problem finding clothes that still fit her. I'll have to get her some new slacks.

March 20th: We went with my cousin to have lunch in a so-called German restaurant in Bristol. The conversation was mainly about family affairs and Anita was mostly detached.

She perked up when I described her home village in the Alps, but when the lunch check came, she scowled at the waitress and said "Das war kein Deutsches Essen." (That was not German food.) She was right about that.

March 28th: While I was busy at the computer, Mollie went down for the mail and left the door open. Anita walked out and down to the car. She found the door locked and came back to sit in the lobby. Mollie found her and I took them both to shop for new slacks, then to Anita's nail salon, before going to our favorite tavern for lunch.

That afternoon we sat at the balcony and watched the birds peck at their seed. Her two doves were the only birds that did not fly away when she made a hand motion. I asked if she had given them names. She smiled. "No, not yet."

That night we went to see the TAO Drummers. Anita was transfixed by the performance and drummed on the dashboard all the way home. I dug out my old blues harmonica and played some of her favorite Swiss folk tunes before she dropped off to sleep in her chair.

April 6th: Went to the fitness club and the coffee shop for Anita's bagel and cream cheese and she was more attentive to her surroundings than usual. I was encouraged and decided to take her to visit my cousin in Barrington. When we arrived, she stayed only a few minutes before returning to the car. I told my cousin not to be upset. "It's no reflection on you, just an annoying manifestation of Anita's condition."

April 11th: This was a trying day. Anita would sit still for only an hour before putting on her coat to stand at the door. It was not possible for me to get any writing done, so I took her to a local Indian restaurant for dinner.

April 22nd: We drove to Vermont on the 18th to spend a few days with my daughter and her family. Anita was relaxed after a dose of tranquilizers and remained so for the four-hour trip. She brightened up immediately when she saw the grandchildren and it was evident the trip had been worthwhile.

She kissed and hugged the two smallest grandchildren and nodded with a smile when she was shown crayon drawings they said were made just for her. It was satisfying to see her relaxed when around small children.

We stopped for a meal on the way home. While I was in the restroom, Anita left the table and went back to the car. When I brought her back inside there were plenty of curious looks from the other customers. I couldn't tell them she feels uncomfortable in strange places or that her anti-anxiety pills don't always help.

April 30th: The past ten days have been challenging and with little optimism. Her wandering has caused me anxiety and worry about her safety. Last week, while I was talking to a sales clerk at the Warwick Mall, she wandered off into the crowd and it took fifteen minutes to find her in the main corridor heading for the parking lot. One of my neighbors suggested I buy a dog leash to keep her close. I crossed that idea off—it is degrading and unthinkable.

I took her to New York City on the bus last week and we saw a Broadway musical and did some shopping at Macy's for a new summer outfit. I took her to her favorite hair dresser for a new hairstyle and that night she was in a good mood. She smiled and was responsive to an old colleague of mine and his wife while we had dinner at one of our most favorite places, Gallagher's Steak House. For some reason, she refused to eat her meal and just sipped on her wine. I had to explain that this was one of the phases of her condition and was no reflection on them. Our friends were kind and sympathetic.

She wandered off at the supermarket in Lincoln two days ago and I couldn't find her. I went nuts for an hour until a policeman called. He told me she had been found a half mile away walking along the highway shoulder. I picked her up and the rescue personnel were polite, understood my situation, and advised me to keep her within eyesight whenever we were at the mall.

May 2nd to 20th: An x-ray showed that the spot on Anita's lung has receded, but she continues to have coughing spells. She needs attention when getting dressed, putting on her makeup, and combing her hair and has started rubbing her palms together while on the toilet or at the table. She won't stop until she hears them squeak. I don't know why she does it.

She interacts in a friendly manner at the fitness club, but her verbal connections are limited. I stopped giving her the prescribed anti-anxiety pills, but will restart if she shows need.

I sit with Anita for long sessions coaxing her to talk about her old friends in Pontresina and of the many walks we made in the alpine valleys. She listens and smiles, sometimes responding with a few words. I can see her longing to be home again in the Alps—and I long to be there with her.

May 30th: It rained, so we sat on the couch and watched her favorite TV westerns. When birds came to the balcony, she waved and smiled. When I stood up, they flew away. She shook her head in reprimand and I promised they would return.

June 30th: This has been a demanding and weary month. Two of my daughters came for Father's Day and were upset when they saw Anita's condition. They worried about the strain on me, but I assured them I was very able to do what is needed for her care. I explained that Anita was able to do small chores. She washes the dishes but forgets where the cutlery goes and that I had found silverware in the trash. I said I have to look through the trash can every day before I take it out to the dumpster and they shook their heads in sympathy.

Almost all my time this month was spent cooking and cleaning, as well as looking to her personal needs. A local woman comes in twice a week to help with cleaning and laundry. She is very thorough and gets along well with Anita.

Anita has a weak bladder and has to be changed each morning. I put her into Depends underpants and have put an absorbent pad on the bed as well.

Took her to the neurologist for a checkup and he said Anita was in the fourth stage of Alzheimer's. I did not have to be told that—it was obvious. My own research made me aware of each stage of progression. The visit was a waste of time and money.

Found a trained caregiver for Anita—hope she is good.

July 31st: Anita's caregiver, Sophia, is working out well. She is strong and knows the ropes.

Anita is having bowel control problems now and has to be changed once or twice each day. Sophia handles the problem well.

Sophia took Anita to the zoo at Roger Williams Park for a ride on the carousel with some small children. She told me Anita smiled and waved to all the children during her time in the park and I told Sophia of Anita's love for small children and how involved she was in the children's hospital in Zurich.

Our routine at the fitness club continued and Sophia went along to watch Anita. She went with us to lunch at the tavern, anticipated Anita's needs, and I am grateful for her help. It has given me time for my writing.

December 21st: There was continued downward trend in Anita's condition this year. On the few days when she seemed better, our hopes were always dashed when she slipped to a lower level of awareness. I knew there would be periods of stability and that they would be temporary. My heart is heavier each time I look into her beautiful eyes and know I can't help her.

I took Anita to Vermont for Christmas to see my daughter, her children, and grandchildren. She was relaxed in the car after the anti-anxiety pills took effect. We stayed at the Shire Motel in Woodstock. Anita had stayed there on earlier trips and loved the view of the river and the fact that she had her own king-size bed.

When we arrived at the farm, Anita kissed and hugged each of the children and each child returned her affection with kisses, smiles, and hugs.

After a big lunch, Anita went outside to watch the children having a snowball fight. She headed down the driveway toward our car and slipped on the ice, fell hard on her face, and badly gashed her eyebrow and lower lip.

We loaded her into my car and my grandson and his friend held her in the back seat while we rushed to the town clinic. The town clinic was closed for the day so we drove twenty miles to Dartmouth hospital in New Hampshire. She was checked for a concussion before she received eight stitches in her brow and six in her lower lip. There was no concussion.

When we got back to the farm, her eyes were glazed, but she did not seem to be in pain. She received full attention from everyone until we left for home the next day.

The doctor who stitched her up was very talented and a week later when the dressings were removed, there were only minimal scars. I thank him for that.

PART V

Chapter Nine

THE BURDEN OF DESPERATION

The late stages of Alzheimer's disease differ from case to case and you cannot, in good faith, cast each sufferer in a common mold. Each beloved victim deserves love and care as a unique person.

Placing a loved one with Alzheimer's in an institution should be the last and most extreme resort. Such a decision should not be determined by the time and effort necessary to keep your loved one in the safety of his or her home. In most cases, he or she has devoted more time and love to raising and caring for you. In the end, by having returned some of that love and care, your life as their caregiver will be made fuller.

* * *

January 2015: The scars on Anita's lower lip and eyebrow have healed well and are barely visible. She no longer recoils when looking in the mirror. I am not sure she remembers her fall at the farm in Vermont and what she endured that day.

Getting her to eat is a problem. She sits and toys with her food, must be coaxed to put it in her mouth and will eat her meat or fish only if it has been cut in small pieces. Every meal is balanced and includes beef, veal, fish, or chicken, vegetables, a salad, and fruit. Every two weeks I make a pot of beef as I did for her at home in Switzerland.

She has always been a fan of my baking, so I make her fudge brownies, oatmeal cookies, and an apple or pumpkin pie. She gets at least one piece of her favorite Lindt chocolate and occasionally a wedge of Toblerone.

I had her teeth checked to see if there was anything to account for her not wanting to chew her food. All was okay. She doesn't seem to enjoy her food as she once did. My Alzheimer's research shows a loss of taste is not uncommon. I have to accept it and continue to make her food tasty.

Anita's part-time caregiver, Molly, left us to take a full-time job, but I was able to hire an experienced nursing assistant with ten years' experience caring for Alzheimer's patients. Her name is Linda and I hope Anita takes to her—I need some time for my writing.

February: This has been a tough month. Cold and heavy snow kept me from taking Anita to the tavern for lunch or for a change of scenery. Linda was out with the flu for four days and I did the washing, dressing, and feeding. It made me appreciate more what Linda has to do for my beautiful princess.

Anita walks to the balcony window each morning to see if I have put out seed for her feathered friends. When she sees them at the seed, she smiles, then sits in her chair for a while to watch her birds come and go.

The weather cleared for a few days so I shopped for food and supplies. It has been difficult to find things Anita will eat. She usually won't eat all of her meal, so I've been giving her a chocolate-flavored energy drink that Linda recommended. I like it myself—it's tasty, but who knows what benefit it will provide.

March: Anita has taken well to Linda and no longer resists standing in the tub for a shower. Her clothes consciousness remains, and she selects what she will wear each day. Linda is impressed by Anita's large wardrobe.

She has adopted the south-end of the sofa, rather than her easy chair, as her seating preference and has a direct view of the balcony, the comings and goings of her bird friends, and her favorite TV programs.

When weather permits, Linda takes her for a walk in the nearby park. There is a small beach the children use in the summer and Linda says Anita enjoys the outing.

"She walks with her head up as though looking for someone or something to appear along the way. Do you know what that might be?"

"Linda, I think she expects to see large white swans like those that populated the Lake Zurich shore when we walked there. She often said the swans owned the lake and would confront people feeding bread to the swans. She would ask them to use only the feed listed on signs posted along the lake."

April: I have been taking Anita to Cricket's lounge for a light lunch during the week and she is at ease with the regulars we have known for four years and they like her. She can handle the lunch special of a half sandwich and a cup of soup and drinks her pint of Stella Artois beer like a trooper.

Our friends enjoy her Swiss accent and ask me why I don't have an accent after having lived in Switzerland for over forty years. I tell them it doesn't always come with the territory. They ask about our favorite foods, so I describe the geschnetzles mit roeshti (wine sautéd veal strips with a pancake of shredded potato) and describe the famous Zurich Kalbsbratwurst and buerli (a veal sausage with a hard crust swiss bread roll). Anita's eyes brighten when I describe the local Swiss foods.

We go to Aiden's Pub in Bristol on Saturdays and I tell Linda about the villages around Lake Zurich where we roamed on weekends. I told her we had looked forward to making a home in America to explore more of this beautiful country, but I ended on a somber note.

"Sadly, it has not turned out as we expected, but we will make the best of each day we have together—come what may."

May and June: With Linda's help, I have had time to go food shopping, work out at the fitness club, do the household bookkeeping, and continue my book writing.

Anita has lost weight and is less aware of what is going on around her. It is discouraging, but predicted.

Linda stayed with Anita four days in June while I went to Michigan to attend my grandson's high school graduation. I returned with presents from everyone in the family and she opened them like a child at Christmas.

Anita had behaved very well and Linda said she didn't seem to notice my absence. That made me feel a little sad.

Her awareness continues to deteriorate and the most disturbing thing is the blank stare she gives me when I talk to her and it takes her a few seconds to recognize me, but when she does, she smiles. Sometimes, when we watch TV, she leans over and gives me a kiss on the cheek—it almost brings me to tears.

The weather now permits short walks in the town park across the road to watch the children play. Her eyes never leave them.

July and August: Anita had a health checkup and her heart and lungs were found normal. Her anxiety pill was changed and proved better. She is less nervous and the sundown wanderings have stopped.

Before she leaves, Linda gets Anita ready to sit with me to watch TV until I put her to bed. Usually, she sleeps until Linda arrives to wash, dress, and make her breakfast.

These two months have been hot and humid and depressing for us all. The beaches on the south shore are very crowded and the traffic on all routes is excessive. My car's cooler struggles to make the environment livable. Given the care necessary for Anita, we can't reach the beach early enough to find a parking place. An alternative had been to take her to the small pool in the apartment complex, but we found the pool to be unclean and went only once. We take her to the little beach in the town park across the road, but she refuses to go in the water and sits on a park bench to watch the kids play and swim. When we leave for home her smile fades. She is clearly glum when the children are out of her sight.

Anita is eating better, has lost some weight, and some of her clothes fit again. She is quicker to recognize the people at the tavern and the neighbors in our apartment building and that's a good step up from where she was two months ago—I hope it lasts.

Linda and I play hand games with her—the hand games she liked to play with my grandchildren in Vermont. She uses the empty hand towel roll as a telescope and watches her bird friends peck at their feed on the balcony. I try to imagine what she is thinking, but she is lost in the shadow of a child's world that denies me entry.

I had a physical checkup and was told I was in reasonably good shape, but my bald spot is getting bigger—they say you can't have everything.

Linda was happy to hear about my health and reminded me that in case of an urgency she is only twenty minutes away. On her day off, she calls me to check on how we are doing. Her care for both of us is much appreciated.

September: Anita's younger sister, Trudy, flew into Boston from Zurich for a short visit. I had worried that she would not recognize Trudy but was surprised and relieved when Anita smiled, reached out, and embraced her sister as she walked in the door.

Trudy was upset when she saw Anita in her wheelchair and I took her aside to explain her sister's condition and the ultimate prognosis. I confessed my guilt at having taken her away from Zurich and her favorite haunts and many friends. She tried to console me.

"Parigi, I know how much you love each other and how much pain you must be having, but I know she could not have more loving care than she has with you. Everyone back home will be praying for you both and some miracle cure."

We went out twice for dinner at our favorite restaurant and Anita ate her favorite dishes with only a little help from Linda and myself. She smiled as Trudy, Linda, and I talked and nodded her head at mention of names she remembered. My sadness returned when Anita's eyes clouded as her sister left.

November 23rd: When Linda got Anita out of bed and dressed, her skin was clammy and she was unstable. The left side of her face and mouth were drooping and we thought she may have had a stroke. We took her to a nearby hospital where she had a brain scan and a series of tests. We were told she would remain overnight until the tests were analyzed. If the findings permitted, she would be released next morning.

Linda volunteered to stay with Anita, keep me informed and would bring her home when released. The whole situation had me on pins and needles until the word came that there was no evidence of her having had a stroke.

At home, Linda told me Anita had not been well cared for. The nursing staff was inattentive, she was fed only one meal and they had to be reminded several times to bring her something to drink. The episode convinced me to take her to the Miriam Hospital in any future emergency.

The episode reminded me of how superior the Swiss hospitals and medical care were. Once again I felt the guilt of having taken Anita from the place we both loved.

December: We ended the year by decorating our small Christmas tree and sending cards to friends and relatives in Europe and America. We had no visitors, but many calls from friends and relatives around the world. Except for a short visit from three of my grandchildren, Linda was our only company during the holiday season.

We cuddled on the sofa each evening, watched the winking tree lights, and tuned in our favorite TV shows and holiday concerts. I blanked out visions of the future—Anita was the only company I needed to see me into the coming year.

By and large, 2015 was a bummer year for us, but Anita is still with me and that is all that counts—she is my soul mate. I pray for a miracle that will rid her of this horrible and debilitating illness.

PART VI

Chapter Ten

ACCEPTING THE INEVITABLE

The accepted code of morality for most people is that life is a precious endowment to every living creature. To hold otherwise is unthinkable. However, most of us accept that all life, in any form, must someday end.

We accept the end of life as inevitable and when faced with the coming loss of a loved one, we prepare for that day in the most caring and responsible way. In a humane society, to do otherwise is unacceptable, and we accept the mental, physical, and economic costs involved for we deem them burdens of love.

While the shadows gradually fall on a loved one, we provide a daily ray of sunshine. We must provide the light to guide them for they will not have our hand to hold on their way.

* * *

January - March 2016: The heavy snow and cold kept us mostly isolated during January and February and the only ventures Anita and Linda made with me were to Lincoln to do grocery shopping. Anita was always dressed in her fur-lined coat, boots, and wool hat for the shopping and enjoyed roaming the supermarket aisles, hand-in-hand with Linda. After shopping we had our morning treat at the coffee shop. Her order of coffee and a toasted bagel with cream cheese and jelly has never varied since the days at our coffee shop in Zurich. If I forget to order jelly on the cream cheese, she squints.

One day in March Linda took Anita to visit Lena, her infant grandchild. She enjoyed it so much Linda made it a weekly occasion. Anita insisted on holding and playing with Lena during the whole visit and was given one of Lena's dolls as a gift. We named it after Anita's younger brother Thomi. He had passed away the previous year, but Anita had not been told of his passing. She cared for Thomi as an infant so there may be a spark of memory when she holds the doll.

We took Anita to Target and bought clothes for her Thomi doll.

She had poked through the displays, nodded her head to the items she liked and Thomi soon had a new set of clothes.

In mid-March, I learned that my oldest daughter had bone cancer. It was her third bout with cancer and another subjection to dreaded chemotherapy, but my grandchildren said she was not giving up the fight. My daughter Edith was flying in from Colorado to manage a program for her sister's care, and I was somewhat relieved knowing Cynthia would be in good hands during her ordeal. I was now at a new level of mental stress.

I decided to drive to Vermont to assure myself of my daughter's care. Linda stayed with Anita every hour I was away. During the long drive home, my head was filled with images of both Cynthia and Anita and the ordeals they faced in the coming months—it was depressing. I became angry about my inability to bring some salvation to the two women I loved and cherished.

The past two months have shown an increase in Anita's need for personal care. Loss of control over her bodily functions places us on constant alert to assure her cleanliness. Watching her decline is painful.

April: Anita surprised me one day by answering with a clear and distinct "No" when I offered her some sliced apple. It was the first word she had uttered in about a year. A day later, when being awakened from a nap, she opened her eyes and startled Linda by speaking a few words in a clear voice.

"I couldn't understand what she said. It was not in English. I think it was in German. I'm sure you would have understood her."

These two incidents indicated some part of her speech center is able to function. The problem is to find some way to stimulate it. Perhaps I can find a speech therapist to work with her.

May: Anita stumbled and hurt her ankle. We thought it was a bad sprain but an x-ray showed a small fracture, so the doctor put her into an ankle boot for six weeks.

Caring for her while she was in the boot gave us challenges and it bothers me that she cannot tell us when she is in pain. We can see her squint her eyes when she tries to walk and know she feels pain. I bought a walker to help her get around safely and so Linda can take her for short walks down the hallway to keep her active until her ankle heals. When the boot was finally removed, she continued to drag her foot while walking. It gave me more concern.

The doctor examined her and could not account for the foot dragging. He told me to try massaging her ankle. I said Linda was already doing that twice a day.

June: Summer finally arrived. Anita's ankle showed improvement and I am able to take her to Bristol and Colt's Drive for short walks on the bay shore. We sit on our favorite bench at water's edge to watch boat traffic on the bay and talk with people walking their dogs. Small children are usually playing in the grass and Anita waves and smiles as they wave back. We usually spend an hour on the waterfront bench before going to Aiden's for lunch. These pub visits and visits to see Linda's grandchild, Lena, are her two favorite outings.

We take a booth at the pub so she can be discreetly fed by myself or Linda. Anita is usually relaxed and seems to recognize our favorite waitress. The pub staff remembers how Anita was on our visits in earlier years and is always gracious. Small town restaurants seem to retain that characteristic.

July: This was not a good time for Anita. She suffered from skin rashes and pressure welts from laying on her side all night. I bought a bubble mattress for the welts and a new security strap to keep her secure in bed.

In mid-July Anita came down with a urinary tract infection and went to the Miriam Hospital for treatment. Linda and I stayed with her for most of the three days she was there and the hospital staff were caring and attentive the entire time and is at the top of my list of best hospitals.

A human services representative came to our apartment each Thursday to see Anita and I learned that most of the things I had been buying for Anita's care could be provided at no cost through prescriptions. It was unexpected good news.

It became more difficult to maneuver Anita in the bathroom. Getting her on and off the toilet, cleaning, changing, and giving her a shower is becoming a strain on Linda when I am not around, so I bought a special shower seat so she would not have to stand while being washed. It helped a lot. She is more relaxed and less resistant to our efforts to wash her.

I remember how she spent half an hour each night in our shower in Switzerland and how rosy and relaxed she was when she climbed into our big bed. It was like sleeping in a bed of lilacs.

August: We had a series of visits from the hospice nurses who checked Anita's vital signs and general health A physical therapist named Chan, comes three times a week to work on her mobility problems and Anita took to her right way because Chan sings to her in Mandarin as she works. Chan has a good voice and it brings back memories of my days in the Far East. The therapy has helped her mobility and we're able to take her for short walks in a nearby park. Linda takes her for walks up and down the hallway twice a day as well.

Feeding her is still a problem. She doesn't chew her food thoroughly and has difficulty swallowing, so we're putting her food in the blender to liquify it. She likes smoothies made with ice cream and fruit and I keep a supply of her favorite ice cream in the freezer.

September: Anita had a checkup with the doctor. He knows of no way to slow her decline and gave her something to help her hold her urine while she sleeps and put her on a new sleeping pill. We are watching her response with the hope she will sleep longer and be more comfortable.

October: Anita is responding to therapy and is much more mobile. Her system is functioning better and with the TENA wrap-around underpants I ordered on the internet, it's easier for Linda to change her standing up in the bathroom. I see the shame in her face as she goes through the twice-daily requirement of keeping her clean and comfortable and it hurts me more than it does her.

At five o'clock last Sunday, I woke up when I heard a thud and a groan. Anita had slipped off the bed and into the narrow space between our beds. I had to shove the beds apart to have enough space to lift her into a sitting position. My back was not strong enough to lift her to her feet, so I slept with her on the floor with a comforter, blanket, and pillow until Linda arrived to help me get Anita on her feet.

I explained that Anita had somehow removed the safety strap, rolled over and fell out of bed in her sleep. Had she rolled to her right side the safety rail on that side would have prevented her from falling out of bed.

"Anita always sleeps on her right side, Linda. Why she turned on her left side is a mystery."

We saw that she had a bruise on her right hip but didn't seem to be in pain. I will have to find a bed strap she cannot easily remove. She limps when walking—might be pain in her hip.

The days are getting shorter as winter sets in for what promises to be a housebound period of inactivity. That means finding new ways to keep Anita occupied and relaxed until the warm weather returns. I'll make the apartment a happy and festive place for the coming holidays and Linda will help by bringing her granddaughter with her more often. That alone will certainly buoy Anita's spirits.

November: Anita is still mobile and walks in the hallway with Linda every day, but she still drags her right foot. They spend time in the lobby visiting with some of the tenants who greet her with smiles and a hug.

The evening caregiver, Ami, comes in at 4:00 p.m. to walk Anita for half an hour, to make her supper and prepare her for bed. She always has a ready smile when Ami arrives and when she is tucked in bed at 9:00 p.m. I am fortunate to have found two caring women as caregivers for my Alpine Princess.

One of my granddaughters came down from Vermont with Elle, her three-year-old daughter. Anita was in heaven and hugged and cuddled Elle for most of the time she was here. When they left, it was her tearful kiss and final hug for Elle that brought me down. I want to know what goes through her mind on these visits, but I can only guess.

Linda brought two more dolls for Anita and she is rarely without one or two of them on her lap.

I stuffed and roasted a small turkey for Thanksgiving and Anita sat in the kitchen all morning watching the process. She tasted the pumpkin pie mix before it went into the oven. From the look on her face, I thought she may have remembered the holiday feasts we prepared in Zurich each year for our Swiss friends. I hope she did—but will never know.

December: This was a trying month. Getting food and drink into Anita was an ongoing chore for Linda and Ami and I hoped they would not become discouraged. I feared she would become dehydrated or have another UTI, so we had to keep her nourished and mobile. She hadn't had a bowel movement for three days and we were worried. Normally, she would have two movements a day, so this change concerned us. We took her to Miriam Hospital and was found to have an impacted bowel and a possible infection. She was purged, given a new medication and released the same day.

We nursed her intently and within a week she recovered her ability to walk without assistance. Both Linda and Ami were as thankful and relieved as myself.

Linda and Ami were very accommodating over the holiday period and filled in for each other so that someone would always be on duty during the daytime. I fed Anita the evening meals prepared by Linda and sat with her to watch our TV shows, or listen to our favorite concert classics on a CD. I was happy to have time alone with her with no distractions and I could tell her stories of our happy life together. Sometimes she responded with a smile.

I assembled and decorated the Christmas tree and, as the lights twinkled, we watched our favorite concerts. The year-end concert from

Vienna was the favorite we had watched for many years. It always soothed and relaxed her.

This has been another long year away from Switzerland and the loss of an environment we so dearly loved was painful. It saddens me not to know what my princess is thinking. Is she having visions of our life in Zurich and of her childhood in the Alps?

I have surrounded my beautiful wife with as much love and affection a loving husband can bring, but I know it is not enough to protect her from the shadowy world facing her.

A Harvard University neuroscientist has been discovering more about the makeup and causes of Alzheimer's and the role inflammation of the amyloid plaque plays in it. Unfortunately, there has been no noticeable effort by our government to fund the work required to massively expand needed research. That neglect adds to the despondent outlook of the loved ones of victims of this terrible condition. In spite of this despondency, I try to remain hopeful that some form of salvation will help Anita.

PART VII

Chapter Eleven

THE DOWNWARD SPIRAL IN 2017

The year started off badly for Anita. She had another UTI in mid-January but recovered from it by month's end. We are prompted to keep an eye out for signs of dehydration.

I constantly question myself about the amount and quality of care I am providing for Anita—the answer is never satisfying. It is not possible for me to know if she understands the gravity of her condition. I can only assume she does not, and that may be a blessing in itself. I will carry on the fight and will accept the pain and burden of whatever comes.

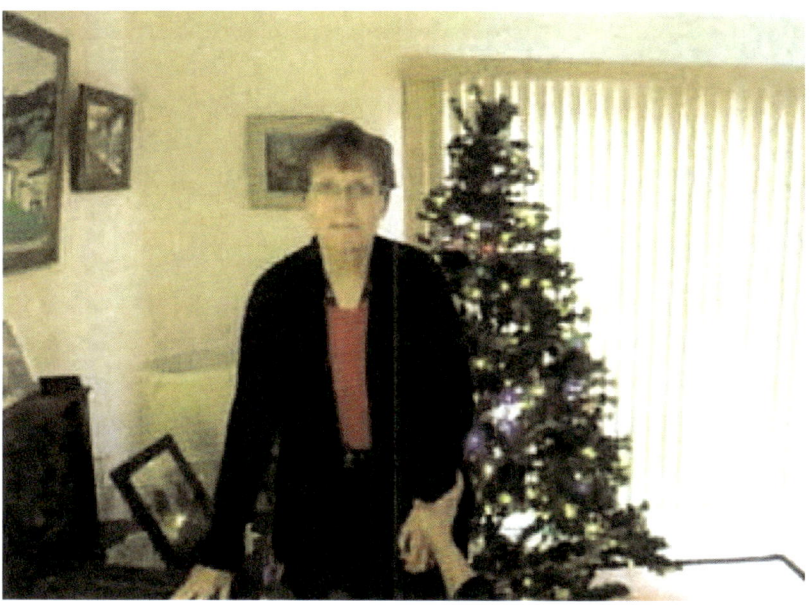

Anita on New Year's Day 2017

January has been without snow, but eventually the. hammer will fall and keep us from getting Anita out to her twice-weekly therapy sessions, and will otherwise screw up our routine.

February: We had a foot of snow by mid-February and it turned very cold. Linda had trouble getting to work in her old klunker. I have to help her trade up to something dependable.

We've found a trick to get Anita to open her mouth for food. We put a slice of apple in her hand and when she opens her mouth we put in her food. The process takes time, but we have patience.

She continues to have trouble walking, and for her first few steps she drags her right foot. We think she has some arthritis in her right knee or hip and will have another x-ray done. It is possible that the damage was more than a bruised knee from her fall off the treadmill at the fitness club. The x-ray taken after her fall may have missed something.

February: At the beginning of the month Anita could not stand or walk and had to be moved in her wheelchair. We were hoping it was temporary, but it persisted and I took her to Miriam Hospital. An x-ray discovered a broken hip and a simple fracture of her upper right arm. The doctor said the hip fracture was not recent, but the arm fracture was.

I could not be sure, but I think the arm damage might have been caused when she fell out of bed and I tried to lift her by grasping her arm. The hip fracture may have happened when she fell from the treadmill and bruised her knee. It is the only possibility I can think of—and it bothers me.

She underwent surgery and received a partial hip replacement. The young surgeon said the operation was successful. His statement later proved incorrect.

Anita was discharged after four days and then moved to a rehabilitation center recommended by the hospital social worker. She was admitted for a two-week stay.

The rehab center was an eye-opener for Linda and myself.

There were about one hundred patients under the care of three registered nurses and one physician. During the two-week period the physician visited Anita just once. Forty patients were housed on Anita's floor and after my insistence, she was assigned one of the two private rooms. There were four nursing assistants and a small staff of minimum-wage workers for forty people on the ward. Linda said there was no way she would leave Anita alone for two weeks in that environment.

Linda stayed with Anita from nine each morning until four and I was with her from three until eight. Linda selected Anita's meals from the limited menu, fed her, and made sure she was kept clean and comfortable. The staff members were thankful for Linda's efforts. They were generally kind and attentive to all the ward patients, but openly acknowledged the understaffing of the center.

The physical therapy staff was young and proved to be of little help to Anita—and the patients in general. We took Anita to the therapy room and found it woefully inadequate for ministering to the needs of the residents. The staff was too cautious when handling Anita and refused to put pressure on her to stand, walk, or do minimal leg exercises. When we wheeled her back to her room, we stood her in the walker and took her for walks in the corridors. She responded well.

After one week of walking in the corridors, Anita was able to use her walker without assistance. She was alert during our strolls around the center and smiled at the staff and patients she recognized. There was an atrium where she could sit to enjoy the sunshine and the scenery and where we could talk with the family members and caregivers of other patients suffering with dementia and Alzheimer's. The caregiver was usually a wife, but a few were husbands, a son, or a daughter. All showed sympathy for Anita and most of them openly shared their caregiving story—often with tears.

I was eager to take Anita home and not have to worry about her care. By the middle of the second week, she was discharged and left the building with a broad smile and a prolonged wave goodbye.

March: Anita is home again and in good spirits. She still needs assistance to walk, but her appetite is much better. We blend and puree all her food so she does not have to chew, and all her meals are nutritious and tasty. I found some organic hemp oil that helps keep her calm and seems to reduce the pain in her hip.

I took Anita to Butler Center to check up on her hip. The surgeon who performed the surgery said it was healing well. I asked if there might have been some nerve damage to account for her inability to walk properly. He said he could see nothing to indicate a nerve problem. I was not surprised by his reply.

April: Anita continues to have trouble walking, drags her right foot, and I can see she has pain in her right knee. Linda massages her legs each evening before putting her to bed. We cannot understand why x-rays of her knee show nothing to account for her discomfort. I bought a knee brace for her, but it hasn't helped.

She sits on the sofa each afternoon with an electric blanket over her knees and watches her favorite television programs. Sometimes I play her favorite operetta songs on my harmonica and then sing her favorite German song, "Edelweiss." She moves her lips to follow and wants to sing along, but taps my arm in time with the music. I am thankful for any response from her, no matter how slight it may seem to others.

My daughter Edith and her husband, Darrell, came in from Colorado for a three-day visit. Anita smiled broadly as Darrell held her hand and I think there was a spark of memory. Anita had often said she was happy Edith had found such a good man and her spirit was notably higher during the visit. She sat with Edith on the sofa and went through photos of their past visits with us in Switzerland. The photo that evoked her greatest smile was one of Anita and my eight-year-old granddaughter, Ella, walking hand-in-hand down a hillside in the ski resort of Arosa. I removed the photo and told Edith to say it was from Anita to her Godchild Ella.

Their departure was heartrending. Anita would not let go of Edith's hand or let go of Darrell's shirt as tears streamed down her cheek. It took a few moments before we could calm her by promising they would both be back soon with Ella. By all accounts offered by the doctors we had visited, her reaction to the visit should not have been emotional. That was not what we had experienced. Perhaps there is more to her memory than we thought.

June: I try not to show Anita, Linda, and Ami how depressed I am, but it is difficult. Each morning I get up, shake the cobwebs from my head, and tell myself to stay strong for Anita.

It's been three months since her hip surgery and no noticeable improvement in her walking. When she stands next to me, she is at least two inches shorter than her former five-foot and eight inches. Her hair is turning gray and Linda says she rubs her temples and shakes her head in front of the bathroom mirror. We will give her a touch of color and watch her reaction.

We started a food program recommended by the Alzheimer's Association and, to our surprise, she feeds herself pieces of fruit after she drinks her blended meal. She is calmer and seems to be more aware of what is going on around her. The visiting nurse from the hospice says her vital signs are normal, but who knows what that means. Linda and Ami are her guardian angels and I am grateful for each day they are with us.

The weather has been good and I will take her to Colt State Park in Bristol. She can sit in her wheelchair to watch the snowy seagulls circle overhead. She waves at children and I savor her every smile.

August: Linda found a pair of Anita's high-shoes in the closet and took her for a walk in the corridor. It was a surprise performance. She walked with a little assistance without dragging her foot. She was animated and smiled broadly at the end of her walk. She will walk in heels from now on.

Anita has coughing spells after each meal and during her first hour in bed. For some reason, even after she has had a drink, she retains some food in her mouth and in her throat. We do not know how to remedy that and her doctor had no suggestions. During her last examination he did not examine her throat for an obstruction and I vowed to find a new primary physician who has not dismissed the needs of patients such as Anita.

I have lost some respect for the US medical profession, at least in the medical practitioners I have been exposed to since coming back to Rhode Island. However, the two medical centers I continue to have high regard for is the Massachusetts General Hospital in Boston and the Miriam Hospital in Providence.

Many senior citizens I know in Rhode Island tell me the value a doctor places on the well-being of older patients is based on the potential for long-term fee income. I hope that's not so.

September: This was a frustrating month. Anita has lost more weight and her doctor has no suggestions for her care beyond those measures we are already taking on a day-by-day basis. After more discussions with family members and with some nearby caregivers of Alzheimer's sufferers, the consensus once again was that a person with short-term life expectancy is not at the top of the primary physician's priority care list. That opinion is worrying.

When I was a small-town boy, the family doctor was a respected and approachable member of the community. He usually had his office at home, often made house visits, and knew much about his patients and their families—a far cry from the modern-day physician. One can see what affect the red tape and cost burdens of working under today's health system has had on patient handling—it means less time for the patient and more time for paperwork. Most physicians will agree with this truth, but remain silent.

October: Cindy, my oldest daughter in Vermont, passed away at the age of sixty-seven. She had suffered through three bouts with cancer. I was with her on her last days and she asked how Anita was doing and I said she was doing as well as could be expected. As I kissed her and rose to leave, she smiled and tightened her grip on my hand. She died that night. My drive home required frequent stops for emotional recovery.

Anita cared for my daughter, her children, and their children, so it was my decision to keep the details of my visit a secret. Linda and Ami were told not to mention it because I did not know how she would react—if at all.

November: Anita's ability to walk has continued to deteriorate and she is confined to her wheelchair for most of each day. Her favorite doll, Thomi, is with her all day and night and she resists any effort to take it from her—even when she is given a shower. When she is out of the shower, she reaches for Thomi and holds him while she is being dressed. She helps Linda put clean clothes on Thomi and smiles happily while it's done. If I could only read her mind, it would ease my own.

Thanks to the spoonful of cannabis oil she gets each night, she is sleeping well.

My grandchildren invited us to Vermont for Thanksgiving. I thanked them but said we would be staying at home. We had a lonely dinner of roast chicken with my cracker stuffing, mashed yams, and homemade cranberry sauce, topped off by Anita's favorite American dessert—warm blueberry pie with ice cream. We drank a glass of our favorite Bordeaux in salute to those who were absent.

We spent the evening cuddling on the sofa and watched some holiday programs. I put her to bed and hummed a few of our favorite songs until she fell asleep.

December: Anita is still losing weight and muscle and has little interest in anything but her Thomi doll and watching her bird friends peck at their seed on the balcony.

We've had no more than an inch of snow so we have been able to make shopping trips for Christmas presents to stuff into small red stockings. When the stockings were filled, Linda pushed Anita around the building to hang one on each apartment door The gesture was well received, and by late Christmas Day, there was a large red stocking on our door with a note saying: "Thank you for thinking of us."

The red stocking episode reminded me of past holidays when Anita took little red stockings to every child in Zurich children's hospital. I like to think it sparked a small memory of those days. It may be too much to expect.

When I finished decorating our Christmas tree, Anita was holding the switch for the twinkle lights. She gazed up at the tree top, smiled broadly, pushed the switch and we all applauded. Many Christmas cards from Europe and America had been hung on a line in the hallway. Anita had read each one with me and had responded with a smile when I read the name of each sender.

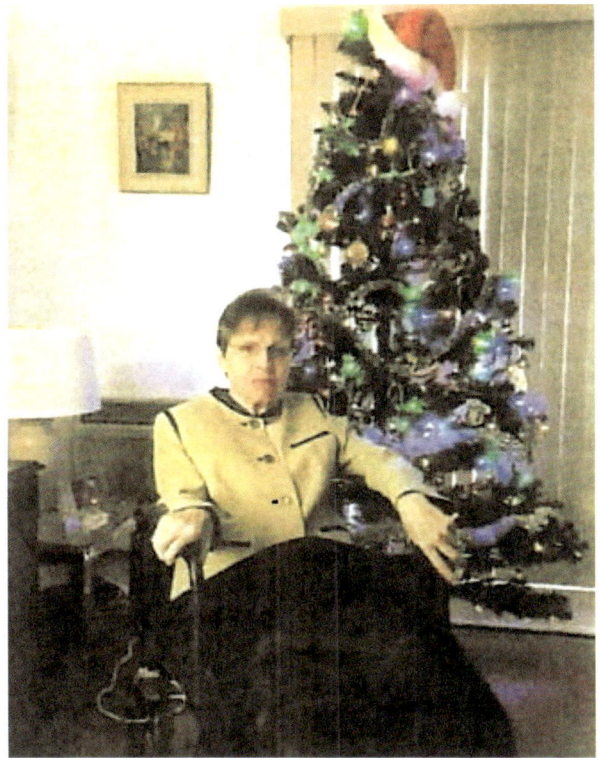

Anita – Christmas day 2017

One of my granddaughters made a visit before flying home to California. She was upset by Anita's condition and tried not to show it until her tears streamed down as she kissed her goodbye for the last time. She promised to say a prayer each night that a cure for Alzheimer's would soon be found for Anita and all the other sufferers of this tragic ailment.

On New Year's Eve, after tucking Anita in bed, I sat and watched the ball fall in Times Square. I hoped it was not another bad omen for us.

As I lay in bed that night, clear recollections of the last year flooded my head. I was becoming more depressed and knew that was not helpful. Now more than ever, Anita needed my full attention and support and I would force myself to be optimistic. She was holding her doll, sleeping peacefully and unaware of my tears. I kissed her cheek and promised this new year would be better.

PART VIII

Chapter Twelve

THE SHADOWS DARKEN

January 2018. The temperature has been in the twenties and a blizzard is forecasted. High winds are predicted and we hope to avoid power outages. We certainly don't need an extra burden. Since we are stuck inside for a while, it means Linda, Ami, and I have to find ways to keep Anita active and occupied.

February: My grandson, Josh, came down from Boston with his four-year-old son, Wyatt—Anita called him "Wyatt Earp." She recognized Josh and Wyatt immediately and sat on the sofa between them to smile through the whole visit. It was sad to see her smile droop as she waved when they walked down the corridor to the elevator.

There were a few sunny days this month, so Linda and I put Anita in the Ford Escape and made a couple of road trips through the countryside. She enjoys riding in the car and seems to recognize places we have often visited—at least we hope she does.

This month she has been going to a local therapist twice a week to exercise her legs and build back some strength. The young therapist is well trained and agrees with me that Anita may have had a slight stroke several years ago. I told her about the 2010 blackout incident in Zurich and that the hospital staff found no indication of a concussion. I confessed it was wrong not having her undergo a brain scan. On the other hand, amyloid buildup in part of her brain may not have begun to show until late 2012, when we began to see something was wrong.

February is the month of international skiing competitions, so we sat together each night to watch the televised events. Anita's eyes brightened when she saw the Swiss flag. Maybe there was a spark of memory of ski runs we made together on our favorite alpine slopes—but who knows? Our many ski outings were so memorable, so vivid, so happy. It is hard to believe they have vanished from her memory

March: In mid-March, Anita came down with a bad cold that kept her awake and coughing. I thought it would put her in the hospital, but to our great relief, she suddenly started to recover. On the downside, my nerves were tattered. It is possible she had an allergy attack and not a flu infection. She has had allergy complications several times in recent years.

At the end of the month, I came down with a bad cold and had to isolate myself from Anita for several days. I stayed out of the apartment most of the day and the caregiving load was put on Linda and Ami until I recovered.

April: The weather for the first half of this month was miserable and we were not able to take Anita outside for some fresh air. Gina pushed her around the building in her wheelchair so she could enjoy seeing some of the residents sitting in the lobby and is always ready to give a warm greeting. She has more difficulty using her walker, so she spends most of their time in the wheelchair, or in her easy chair watching her birds on the balcony. She goes nowhere without her Thomi doll and gets very upset when she is without him.

I get about three to four hours of sleep each night because I get up to check Anita's bed position, check her bed covers and see that she is breathing properly. I may be paranoid from fear that she will forget to breathe in her sleep, so I lay in bed for long periods listening to each breath.

By the end of the month, she was breathing properly and sleeping longer at night. She is not coughing as much and that is a relief. Unfortunately, she has lost more weight and muscular dystrophy has weakened her ability to walk. The twice-weekly visits to the therapist have not helped her condition, and it saddens me when I think of how fit and energetic she was for more than forty years of our marriage.

Once more, the guilt rises when I see her life is not filled with the love of her own children. I was too passive about her self-denial and it will burden me for the rest of my life.

May: We contacted Hope Hospice and had Anita registered, but she will remain at home under our care. A registered nurse will make several visits each week and a social worker will monitor her care and help make an end-of-life plan. My daughter will come from Colorado to help me make plans.

Much of my time this month was spent on the sofa with Anita and thumbing through photo albums dating back to our first meeting in Zurich. She responded to many of the photos with a smile, especially photos of our life in Paris. Those drew her biggest smiles. Our place on Avenue Foch was, of all the places we had lived, the place she loved best.

June: Anita is having bouts of constipation and has to be given laxatives and Linda and Ami monitor and keep her clean. Because there is not enough room in the bathroom to maneuver, they have to change her in the kitchen propped against the table. She is showing no emotion and sits in her wheelchair with her Thomi doll clamped to her chest. The hospice nurse says she has seen many patients in the same condition, but has no advice other than to continue doing what we are doing.

Our prayers bore fruit by the end of the month when she became more responsive, alert, and her appetite improved. Each day with my Alpine Princess is a prayer answered. I can appreciate the pain that other caregivers in this position must bear each day.

July: Anita is a little better and her bodily systems are working again. She is more alert, her appetite has improved, but her ability to stand is very weak. I have to support her while Linda cleans and changes her.

Linda took her to visit her granddaughter Lena on the 4th of July and they had a cookout. When they left for home, Linda said Lena ran to Anita, hugged her, kissed her hand, and Anita gave her a final kiss and smiled as a tear ran down her cheek.

The 4th of July fireworks display in the park across the road was as spectacular as usual and Anita sat at the window with Ami to watch the rockets explode over the trees. I described the Swiss National Day fireworks display in the park above our village and how we sat on the same bench each year. We sang songs with our neighbors, chewed on a bratwurst, and drank beer. Ami said Anita might be remembering something of those times. We put her to bed and she lay on her right side, gazing up at her favorite nightly companion—the portrait of a little girl in a white dress and in her mother's shoes. She flinched at the bang of a rocket but was soon asleep.

August: Anita's muscles are so weak she can no longer walk and spends all day in her wheelchair with her doll. Linda takes her out for a ride in Lincoln Woods twice a week. Getting her in and out of my Ford Escape is too difficult, so we use Linda's smaller Toyota, which has room for her wheelchair. When the weather cools, we will be able to take her to Colt State Park in Bristol for lunch—her favorite outing with me.

Ami has taken a month off to visit her relatives in Senegal and I have hired a nursing assistant, Anair, to fill in. She is from the Cape Verde Islands, and lives a short distance away. Anita has taken well to her—we measure that by the number of times Anita holds her hand and smiles.

By the second week of August, Anita was able to stand to be changed and washed. This is a big improvement, but would not amount to much to an outsider.

The heat has been oppressive and it is necessary to sit her near the air conditioner vent for most of the day. We give her all her favorite drinks to keep her hydrated, but she cannot stay awake for more than an hour before falling asleep and naps for half an hour.

August 16th: Anair came with her six-year-old son this evening and Anita perked up at the sight of him. He is a lively bundle of energy and asked questions about the paintings hanging on our walls. He asked about the painting of Anita's family hotel and shook his head in wonder when told it was where Anita was born in Switzerland. When he was told the girl in the red costume was Anita as a young girl, he walked to her, looked up into her face, and said, "Wow!" I gave him a children's book and he insisted on reading her a story. She couldn't take her eyes off him. When it was time for bed, she reached out and held the boy's hand one last time. As Anair wheeled her down the corridor he shouted, "I hope you have a nice sleep, Switzerland."

Once again, being in the company of a young child was therapy for Anita. I asked Anair to bring her boy again some time. "Your boy is Anita's smile factory."

I searched the house for some small present from Anita to the boy and found an old checker set. I said I would teach him how to play the game when he came again to see Anita.

August 17th, 2018: Anita's coughing woke me, so I turned her on her right side so she could breathe better. My chest tightened and I started to panic when I saw her chest and nightgown were soaked in a dark phlegm. She seemed to be breathing normally, so I propped her up on pillows while I took off her nightgown, washed her and put her in a fresh gown. I held her in my arms and talked to her for over an hour until Linda arrived.

Linda washed her again and put her in clean clothes for breakfast. She was calm and responded to our care with an occasional smile and wave of her hand.

We hoped Anita's coughing had been a temporary lung congestion, but as a caution, Linda called the hospice nurse, told her what had happened and asked that she come and examine her. The nurse said she would arrive before noon.

Anita was resting on her bed and breathing normally when the pharmacy called to say her prescriptions were ready. The pharmacy and the bank were only five minutes away so I told Linda I would go to both places and be back in under an hour. She was to call me if there was another emergency.

I looked for a Swiss chocolate treat at the pharmacy and found the one Anita liked the most—she didn't have to chew it and it melted in her mouth.

It was eleven when I walked in the apartment door and heard Linda calling for me to come to the bedroom. She was sitting on the bed with Anita in her arms, rocking back and forth with tears running down her face.

"She's not breathing right! I don't know what to do!"

I held them both in my arms and we lay Anita down for the last time. Her eyes opened to me, she smiled one last time, and passed into an edelweiss covered meadow that lay above her beautiful childhood home in Pontresina. I consoled Linda.

"Be happy for her. She'll have no more pain. She's at home in her beloved Swiss Alps with the little girl in the white dress who slept next to her each night. Believe me, she will never be alone."

Linda brushed Anita's hair and arranged her clothes before the hospice nurse arrived to write the report on her passing.

I called my daughter in Colorado, gave her the sad news and she said she and her husband would catch the next available flight to be with me.

I sat at her side and waited for the hearse to arrive and my tears fell on her hand as I whispered her favorite song.

"Edelweiss, edelweiss, each morning you greet me,
Small and white, clear and bright, you look happy to meet me.
Blossom of snow, may you bloom and grow,
Edelweiss, edelweiss, bless my homeland forever."

IN MEMORIAL

A memorial service was held for Anita on August 23rd, 2018 and attended by Paris's family members, some friends from the fitness club, and other locals who remembered Anita.

Two of Paris's daughters carried Anita's ashes to her sister in Zurich to be buried alongside her parents and sister at the small hillside church in Pontresina village. Her gravestone was cut from the mountainside next to the home where she spent her youth.

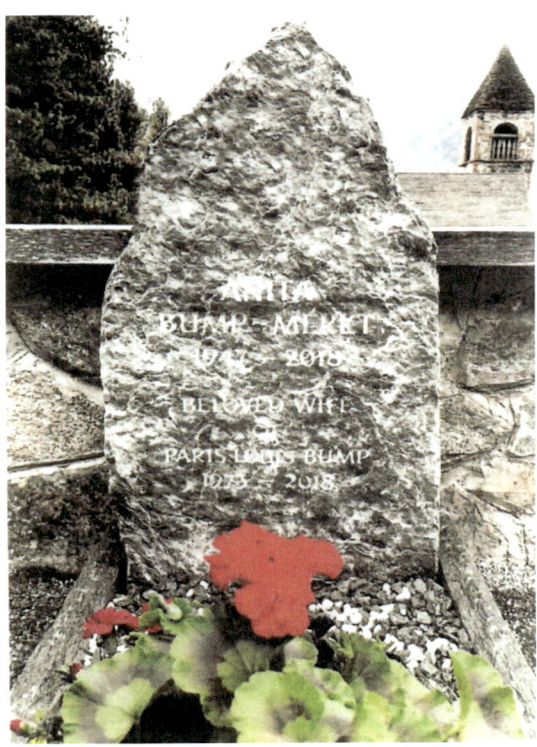

A-1

ADDENDUM

NECESSARY ITEMS AND SUPPLIES FOR PATIENTS WITH ALZHEIMER'S

The following list of items are not all-inclusive and may not fit the needs of all Alzheimer's patients. They were the items used as depicted in this book.

Security:

• Exit doors should be fitted with a device that cannot be operated by the patient. The bathroom door used by the patient should not be fitted with an inside lock—the caregivers should be able to enter in case of emergency.

• Stove controls should be removed when not in use. (Patients, during the sundowner and later stages, often try to use the stove without supervision and can be injured or cause a fire.)

• Bed rails should be in place to prevent falling out of bed. A hospital bed can be rented as an alternative.

• Shower seats should be used to prevent falling when the patients is being washed.

• Sharp items such as scissors and cutlery should be kept out of the patient's reach.

• Medications should be kept out of sight and out of reach by the patient.

• Caustic items such as Lysol, insect spray, rat poison, and all toxic items should be kept out of reach.

A-2

Hygiene:
• Bed strap can be placed under the mattress to cinch the patient and prevent rolling over and falling out of bed. The strap is Velcro ends and adjustable.
• Bubble mattress: An air bubble mattress can be purchased on the internet to prevent bed sores or pressure bruises and help the patient sleep more comfortably.
• Underwear that is padded and absorbent can be used when the patient becomes incontinent. These are readily available with automatic re-order through TENA on the internet. They are much less costly than similar items available at the pharmacy.
• Body lotions to avoid skin dryness should always be applied after the patient is bathed. Lotions are available to prevent bed sores.
• Absorbent bed pads can be purchased and placed under the bedsheet to protect the mattress.
• Surgical gloves should be used when changing the patient and are available at low cost at any surgical supply store,
• Washable Bibs of waist length are available at any surgical supply store and should be used when feeding the patient.
• Electric tooth brush: A rotary toothbrush should be used after each meal if there is a problem to get the patient's mouth open for a conventional brush.

A-3

Walking aids:
• Walker – A four-legged walker with two wheels and two stilts will assist the patient's mobility and balance.
• Wheelchair – Adjustable wheelchairs can be purchased or rented at any surgical supply store. It should be collapsible for easy transport in the car trunk.